In The Future Everyone May Eat Better But You Can Start Now!

More than a half-century ago, pioneers such as Otto Carqué were warning—in terms that sound strangely familiar today—of the decline in the quality of our diet and life, of the rise in processed foods, of the abandonment of sound natural nutrition, the increase in degenerative diseases, the ecologic and health dangers of our mania for meat.

Now, unhappily, disease is dramatically on the rise, the quality of foods falls year by year, and the end of an over-abundant supply of meat is in sight. *Otto Carqué's warnings have come all too true!*

But *Vital Facts About Foods* is more than prophecy; it shows how each reader can take his own and his family's nutrition in hand and, at maximum gain in health and a significant saving in cost, eat for the greatest well-being and enjoyment. Thorough analyses of all foods, and suggested recipes and menus make it possible for even someone completely uninformed about nutrition to understand what sound nourishment is and why it is necessary.

OTTO CARQUÉ'S

Vital Facts About Foods

Keats Publishing, Inc. New Canaan, Connecticut

Dedicated
to my dear wife,
Lillian,
who through her sincere and earnest
spirit of cooperation
has greatly assisted the author
in his work of
food reform.

Otto Carqué's VITAL FACTS ABOUT FOOD

Published in 1975 by Keats Publishing, Inc.

ISBN: 0-87983-113-8
Library of Congress Catalog Card Number: 75-18697

Printed in the United States of America

PIVOT HEALTH CLASSICS are published by
Keats Publishing, Inc.
36 Grove Street, New Canaan, Connecticut 06840

CONTENTS

PART I

The Food Question in All Its Aspects

PART II

Practical Dietetics

PREFACE TO THE THIRD EDITION

It is with emotions mingled with satisfaction and sympathy that I write the preface to the third edition of VITAL FACTS ABOUT FOODS. Satisfaction—that the second edition has again been exhausted with astonishing rapidity and that it has enjoyed the same enthusiastic reception as that accorded its maiden appearance. Sympathy—because of the untimely demise of the author who suffered fatal injuries in an automobile accident a year and a half ago.

The avalanche of tributes paid to him in memorial meetings and writings has forcefully impressed me, his widow, with the sacred trust of his unfinished tasks and with the great responsibility of amplifying his scope of useful activity in matters appertaining to rational nutrition, health and disease.

While I consider my literary efforts puny as compared with the scholarly achievements of the author's masterful pen, I nevertheless will exert every effort to pass on to suffering humanity the benefits of latest facts, developments and discoveries in the realm of scientific food research and Orthopathy, i. e., the lawful and orderly adjustment of the internal and external relations of the organism.

Lillian R. Carqué

July 6, 1936

PREFACE TO THE FOURTH EDITION

Before releasing the fourth edition of VITAL FACTS ABOUT FOODS, the writer, widow of the illustrious author, has permitted herself the privilege of correcting statements presented or conclusions promulgated by the author that later facilities of research have found at variance with current accredited nutritional knowledge. These corrections have been commented upon either by means of foot-notes, or deleted entirely and replaced by new material, revealing up-to-date information and discoveries ascertained through recent nutritional research. These facts are advanced with no intention of treating irreverently the late Otto Carque's dietetic masterpiece, but rather to supplement such findings as could not be proved to his satisfaction at the time of his conscientious probings with the facilities, laboratory technique and other scientific information then available to him.

Lillian R. Carqué

February, 1940

PREFACE TO THE ELEVENTH EDITION

Since Otto Carqué wrote this book, many individual books have been written about one or another of the principles he set forth. Refined carbohydrates, aluminum, salt, highly concentrated meat diets, additives in foods or chemicals on them, all have often played the roles of villains. Just as the heroes' parts have been taken by vitamins and minerals, the proper proportion of foods in combination, composition and amounts, nut milks, soybeans, raw foods—all familiar to us now. But the astounding fact about this book is that they are all together, as feasible now as they were long ago. We are proud to present this new time-honored edition.

Keats Publishing, Inc.
September, 1975

PREFACE

Fifteen years ago the author, who has made the study of foods and nutrition and their relation to health and disease his life work, published a comprehensive volume, entitled RATIONAL DIET, which was followed by NATURAL FOODS—The Safe Way to Health, and the KEY TO RATIONAL DIETETICS. In all these treatises special attention was paid to the mineral elements or organic salts in foods and to their great value in the maintenance of health and in the prevention of disease.

As these books are now out of print, the author has decided to concentrate the essentials of these three books, together with much added information, into *one volume* entitled *VITAL FACTS ABOUT FOODS.* This book will give the student of dietetics a comprehensive knowledge of the latest discoveries in the fields of food chemistry and nutrition and in their application to the daily life. Fortunately our schools and colleges are beginning to pay more attention to the subject of rational diet and its relation to health according to the latest findings of biochemistry. The teaching of dietetics, especially in regard to the rational preparation and combination of foods, is a long step forward in the right direction.

Notwithstanding the remarkable progress that has been made in the science of nutrition for the last thirty years, diet-reform is progressing slowly. We are living in an age of commercialism and millions of dollars have been invested in the manufacture of demineralized and devitalized food products, for which a large demand has been created by shrewd, misleading advertisements often supported by statements of chemists, evidently hired for the occasion. The general public, devoid of exact knowledge concerning food values, buys these impoverished products, unaware of the fact that they undermine health and vitality.

It is now an acknowledged fact that our physical and mental well being largely depends on the normal alkalinity of the blood, while acidosis or toxemia is the primary cause of nearly all pathological conditions. Few realize that quick elimination of the body's waste poisons is a most essential factor in nutrition. If the alkalinity of the blood is lessened, digestion, assimilation and elimination suffer. A thorough understanding of food values, especially of the chemical composition of foods in regard to their mineral contents is, therefore, indispensable.

The influence of the conditions of the mind on the physiological functions of the body should not be underestimated. But, on the other hand, it cannot be gainsaid that the former are often affected to some degree by our dietetic and hygienic habits and the condition of our internal organs. The influence of food and diet on public health and morals has been and will always be an important factor in the progress and welfare of the human race.

The building of a sound and healthy body and mind should only be a means to an end. It should enable us to discharge our duties more efficiently toward ourselves and our fellowmen. Higher states of society require better men. And by making the unit of society—the individual man—strong, healthy and self-reliant through the adoption of saner methods of living and a higher mental and moral conception of life, we shall make one of the greatest strides toward a new and better civilization.

Lasting reforms can never be brought about by parliaments or sumptuary laws. They must come through individual effort and betterment, based on a deeper understanding of the great regenerative and healing forces of nature which are always active throughout the organic world. Legislative measures may accomplish much in bettering our conditions, but *the only true and lasting reform is that which is wrought within ourselves.*

The present time marks the dawn of a new era in the evolutionary march of the human race. Out of the darkness of the ages where fear and superstition, greed and selfishness held their sway, there gradually comes the awakening of a higher consciousness and the cognizance of the great potentialities of man, under a system of social and economic justice.

To all progressive and unprejudiced thinkers it becomes clear that the universe is not at the mercy of blind forces, but is governed by unchangeable laws, and that the phenomena of life and growth are the result of the wonderful and inimitable creative chemistry of nature. The more closely and conscientiously we live in harmony with nature's laws, the sooner we hasten the coming of a higher order of society characterized by the reign of intellect, universal peace and welfare of all.

With the increasing knowledge of our actual position in nature, we may hopefully look forward to the time when an age of temperance, an age of sanitary reform, an age of plain living and high thinking shall have so regenerated man that he will walk the earth a century and more, carrying out the great law of evolution which culminates in the physical, mental and spiritual perfection of the human race.

Los Angeles, California, September, 1933.

Otto Carqué

PREFACE TO THE SECOND EDITION

VITAL FACTS ABOUT FOODS has been gratifyingly acclaimed both by the laity and the progressive members of the medical profession. The astonishing rapidity with which the first edition of this book has become exhausted, testifies to its great popularity and usefulness as an authoritative guide in the realm of rational nutrition and scientific food research. From letters of appreciation received, may I be permitted to quote the opinion of one of the leading food experts of the United States: "Your work is readable and popular, yet exceedingly thorough and painstakingly accurate. It is by far the best book in the field that I have seen."

I am firm in my conviction that our practical daily application of the fundamental laws of life and health, such as briefly outlined in this present volume, will be conducive to a sense of greater physical well-being and will alleviate markedly many of the world's bodily ills.

Los Angeles, California,
November, 1934

Otto Carqué

PART I

THE FOOD QUESTION IN ALL ITS ASPECTS

CHAPTER I

THE URGENT NEED FOR FOOD REFORM

The first part of the twentieth century will be known, in all probability, as one of the greatest transitional periods in human history. We have recently emerged from a great catastrophe, the World War, which has uprooted many of our cherished traditions and may, in time, completely revolutionize human thought and action. There is no doubt that the deeper, underlying causes of that cruel conflict are to be found not so much in general social and economic unrest, as in the highly enervated, neurasthenic condition of "civilized mankind." There are three factors which are undermining the health and vitality of nations: our enervating system of commercial competition; the increasing consumption of stimulants, narcotics (drugs, tobacco, coffee, tea, alcoholic beverages); and last, as probably the most important factor, a degeneration of ideals coupled with perverted thinking and ethics, with faulty and inadequate feeding during all periods of life following in its wake.

Perhaps there is no field of human thought in which error has been more persistently upheld by acquired habit and education—and often with the direst consequences—than that of human nutrition. There has been a slight improvement in the selection of our foods, indicated by the gradual increase in the consumption of fresh fruit and vegetables within the last ten years; yet many wrong dietetic habits persist, laying the foundation of chronic diseases and of premature death.

An abundant food supply does not necessarily protect man from the effects of wrongly prepared and denatured foods. We know that the average individual eats more than he really needs, while the balance clogs his system with waste matter. The American people now spend over twenty billion dollars every year for food, a large part of which is artificially and wrongly prepared, devitalized and adulterated—certainly a great economic waste.

Enormous amounts of valuable mineral elements or organic salts are lost in the manufacture of white flour, refined sugar, etc.; in the irrational preparation of vegetables for the table. As these organic salts are really *"the building stones of the body"* they cannot with impunity be dispensed with, for lack or deficiency of any of these elements in our food in time causes serious disturbances and ultimately wrecks the human organism.

Nearly all diseases that have baffled the medical profession may be helped by a corrective diet, and it may be truthfully said, that many human ailments are traceable to insufficient and faulty nutrition. In no part of study and observation has medical need been more inadequately met than in that of rational dietetics, both in relation to the maintenance of health, and in the treatment and prevention of disease. By far the most detrimental effect of faulty nutrition is the result of habitual errors of one kind or another, which are not sufficiently grave to command immediate attention. For instance, we may abuse our pancreas and kidneys for years, without the feeling of pain, until these organs are finally injured beyond repair. It is the gradual operation of more or less constant, but unperceived causes, rather than of accidental exposures to abnormal conditions, which in most cases are responsible for undermining the health of the individual.

At present, after approximately two generations of experience with a diet of white bread, excessive meat-eating, refined sugar, badly prepared vegetables, and excessive use of salt and spices, we are confronted everywhere with malnutrition, especially among children of all ages, faulty bone growth, bad teeth, poor eyesight, curvation of the spine, constipation and the many evils arising from it.

The old and misleading dietary standards are still being upheld by our educational institutions, our magazines and newspapers, and are followed in nearly every family and public eating house. The dietary of most hospitals, reformatories, prisons, and asylums is faulty and needs thorough revision. In most instances the abnormal mental and physical condition of the inmates is aggravated by wrong feeding. These unfortunates require, above other hygienic measures, a carefully selected diet of wholesome, natural foods, containing the necessary elements for purifying and alkalinizing their blood, and for building up their vital resistance. Lack of instruction in rational dietetics, especially preventive feeding, is still the weak point in the system of medicine.

Our physical and mental well-being largely depends on the alkalinity of the blood, while acidosis or *toxemia* is the primary cause of nearly all pathological conditions. Few realize that proper elimination of the bodily waste is a most essential factor in nutrition. Denatured foods cause starvation. Lack of elimination causes poisoning. Death through retention of waste poisons comes faster than that resulting through starvation.

The foundation for a strong and healthy mind and body is laid during early childhood and before birth. Proper nutrition and care, especially during the first years of our existence, are of the greatest importance. If our ideal is a better race physically, mentally and morally, the best that a mother can give her offspring is none too good. And no contribution that a woman can make to society is more vital than that of bearing and raising healthy children. Yet statistics show that the state of health of our coming generation is far from satisfactory.

The chief medical examiner in the schools of Washington, D.C. said that more than 90 per cent of the school children at six years of age have some physical defect.

The United States Board of Education reports that fifteen million children in the United States are in some manner defective. Some have more than one defect. Here are the statistics issued from the United States Board of Education, Washington, D.C.:

400,000 children have organic disease.
1,000,000 children have tuberculosis.
1,000,000 children have spinal curvature.
4,000,000 children are malnourished.
6,000,000 children have enlarged tonsils, adenoids and other gland diseases.
10,000,000 children have defective teeth.
15,000,000 children have need of attention for physical defects.

Fifteen billion dollars is estimated the annual economic loss due to ill health, expense of sickness, hospitals, hospital maintenance, lost wages, inefficiency of workers and premature death.

Heart disease is the chief cause of death in this country and is steadily becoming more destructive. In 1928, in the United States, it caused 237,649 deaths, a rate of 207.7 per 100,000 of population. Pneumonia was next with a rate of 98 and cancer third with that of 95.9. Kidney disease was a close fourth, at 95. Then came cerebral hemorrhage and softening of the brain, 87; next accidents and tuberculosis each 79.2; congenital malformations and diseases of early infancy, 65.6; influenza, 45.2 and diarrhea and enteritis, 26.3.

In nearly all instances it is lack of elimination of the waste poisons aggravated by over-consumption of acid-forming foods which causes premature death. If sufficient alkaline elements are taken daily in the form of fresh fruit and vegetables, a high rate of metabolism—assimilation and elimination—is maintained, long after maturity has been reached. The life-processes will not lose their intensity markedly at the age of 50, if proper attention is paid to biological living, especially to the proper selection and combination of wholesome natural foods and to moderation in quantities. Those who wish to carry their former vigor beyond fifty years and retain health should make a study of foods in their relation to health and disease. There is no doubt that with the application of rational dietetics, man should be able to extend the proverbial three score and ten to five score and ten; and enjoy a happy and useful life at an age which is now considered the limit of man's usefulness.

There is no more fitting conclusion to this chapter than those remarks made by Dr. Robert McCarrison, a renowned English physician.

"There is no subject more worthy of the consideration of those whose life is spent, or to be spent, in guarding national health. It seems to me that in regard to it we have three obvious duties: the first, to instruct the masses as to what to eat and why to eat it; the second, to apply the results of our science to the production of natural foods in abundance and cheap distribution, rather than to the erection of institutions for the treatment of maladies due to their want; the third and most important, ardently to pursue our investigations and the acquirement of knowledge."

There are seven factors which are intimately connected with the normal growth and development of the body, viz.: sunlight, air, water, food, exercise, rest and last, but not least, our attitude of mind. These factors will be briefly discussed in the following chapters.

CHAPTER II

SUNLIGHT, A GREAT THERAPEUTIC AGENT

The Value of Sunbaths

Most important for the preservation of health and vitality are sunlight and air. They are just as necessary for growth and perpetuation of life as are liquid and solid food. "When the sun does not enter, the physician enters," says an old proverb. It has been found that the greatest mortality occurs in the narrow streets of cities and in houses having northern exposures. The inhabitants of southern mountain slopes are stronger and healthier than are those living on the northern sides. Inhabitants of secluded valleys where the sun rises late and sets early, are generally afflicted with peculiar diseases, chiefly due to a lack of direct sunlight and to its salutary power to dissipate and decompose noxious vapors which accumulate in dark and low places.

The sun indeed is the great and ultimate source of all power which manifests itself in the inorganic as well as in the organic world of this planet. Plants require sunlight, above all, for the completion of their complicated organic combinations. While the lowest species of organic life, such as fungi, are capable of developing in darkness, the higher plants which principally support animal life, always depend upon the rays of the sun for the processes of assimilating the elements of soil and atmosphere. They require especially the ultra-violet rays, which we know to be most active in the production of electro-chemical effects. Likewise the animal body is to a large extent directly dependent on sunlight for its growth and healthy development. It is a well established fact that, as the result of an insufficiency of light, the fibrine and the red blood corpuscles become diminished in quantity, while the serum or watery portion of the blood is increased, inducing leukemia, a sickness characterized by a great increase in the number of white blood corpuscles. A total exclusion of the sunlight induces the severer forms of anemic diseases, originating from an impoverished and disordered state of blood.

A frequent exposure of the naked body to the sunlight will greatly assist the system in the performance of all physiological functions. It will especially insure an even distribution of the blood. Such an adjustment of the circulation is necessary for the normal functioning of all organs. People should make it a practice to expose their nude bodies frequently to sunlight and fresh air in order to keep in the best physical condition. Public parks should have enclosures wherein light and air baths can be taken, and these should become an adjunct of every modern progressive city. Sunlight is the best germicide, but it also kills the cells of our bodies, if they are exposed too much to the very intense rays of the sun. Moderation and discrimination should always be exercised. Sunbaths are best taken in the morning, and a room with an eastern exposure should be selected for the purpose.

To start with, a sunbath should last no more than fifteen to twenty minutes. The rays of the morning sun are particularly beneficial. They exert a growth-promoting effect, as well as a disintegrating activity over the poisons in the body by slightly raising the temperature of the blood and tissues.

I am quoting the following paragraphs from Dr. Tell Berggren's excellent book, *"Solar Therapy and Corrective Physical Education"*:

"Before taking leave of the subject of future possibilities of Solar Therapy, it will be well to call attention to a need that must still be met more adequately if our work is to have its full reward: I mean the need which still exists among women and girls for a greater participation in the benefits of the 'sun-kissed' life. In fact, women and girls are in even greater need of this life than the men. It is of still greater importance for them than for the men and boys if we are to overcome rickety tendencies implanted in us through generations of prudery and poor food.

"Our girls and women should be so used to sunshine inside, in the form of sun-radiated food, as well as outside on their naked bodies, that when they later become mothers they would have offspring free from rickety tendencies and the numerous other weaknesses so many now suffer from due to the lack of an intelligent use of the sun. In order to prevent these many weaknesses it is of vital importance that expectant mothers should make full use of the sun during the period of gestation, to be followed by a still more thorough and carefully directed application of the solar rays after parturition while they are nursing their babies.

"While it is now widely recognized that babies should have enough sun-baths or radiant light, according to the season, we feel strongly that sufficient emphasis has not been given to the idea that prospective mothers themselves should also indulge in sun-sports and other similar pleasures. Until this practice becomes more general we cannot expect the race to perceptibly improve. And even when all these things are properly carried out, it will take several generations to offset the damage of the Dark Ages out of which we are now at last slowly emerging.

"The history of solar therapy thus presents a picture of unfoldment, of gradual enlightenment, of slow but sure progress toward general well-being of the race; and from our vantage-point of today we can confidently forecast a future in which all human beings, whatever their caste or their calling, can enjoy the benefits of 'a place in the sun'."

It has also been observed by Dr. Rollier of Switzerland, that deformities of grown people, as well as those of children, have not only been temporarily, but permanently corrected without any other treatment than that of sunlight, artificial ultra-violet light and diet, with proper rest and very simple orthopedic treatment. (See page 90, *Sunlight and Irradiation.*)

CHAPTER III

THE IMPORTANCE OF FRESH AIR

Equal attention should be paid to a continuous supply of fresh air during day and night. Few persons seem to realize the absolute necessity of the electrifying, life-giving oxygen for the maintenance of vitality and the prevention of disease. It has been only a hundred and sixty years ago (1774) when the English scientist, Priestley, and the French scientist, Lavoisier, discovered that we live by means of a chemical process of combustion, by means of which the blood unites with the inhaled air, yielding the products of combustion which we exhale as aqueous vapor and carbonic acid gas. This chemical action corresponds to that which we find in the case of a burning candle or a lamp fed with oil. If the supply of air is cut off we are suffocated, just as the flame of a lamp is extinguished if the air is prevented from passing to it. A man may live more than sixty days without food, and a few days without water, but when deprived of air or oxygen, he dies in a few minutes. This proves that pure air is the most necessary of all the essentials of life.

The Necessity of Proper Ventilation

Atmospheric air consists of two gases, viz.: Nitrogen and oxygen; the former serves only to dilute the oxygen. Besides these two elements the air always contains some aqueous vapor, carbon dioxide and ammonia. On an average, 100 volumes of air contain:

78.35 vol. of Nitrogen
20.77 vol. of Oxygen
0.84 vol. of Water vapor
0.04 vol. of Carbon dioxide
0.0001 vol. of Ammonia
Traces of other gases (ozone, etc.)

There are also various kinds of microbes in the air, depending upon moisture and temperature, causing fermentation and chemical disintegration of organic substances. The composition of air, i.e., its proportions of nitrogen and oxygen, is the same all over the surface of the earth. The degree of moisture or humidity in the air varies according to location and temperature. Carbon dioxide is always present, even in mid-ocean and forest, but its quantity is very small, ranging from three to four parts per ten thousand by volume. In closed rooms, however, where numbers of persons are present and at the same time where coal and gas are burned, the percentage of carbon dioxide rapidly increases. The air also becomes filled with other and more poisonous gases, such as ammonia and albuminoid ammonia, while the amount of oxygen is gradually lowered. The last named factors should be chiefly considered in the proper ventilation of living rooms, schoolrooms, etc.

Many persons sleep with closed windows, because they cherish the old delusion that "night-air is dangerous." After a few hours they begin to breathe the exhaled air over again. In the morning they get up with a tired feeling and have to resort to "eye-openers" which make their condition still worse. It is during the night when we are at rest that the lungs redouble their efforts to inhale life-giving oxygen to recharge the human dynamo. It is therefore even more essential to provide for an adequate supply of pure air during the night than it is in the daytime. There is absolutely no danger of catching cold from cold, fresh air. On the contrary, the bodily heat, which results from combustion, is increased by an abundant supply of oxygen. A cold is really but an effort of the system to cast out impurities, chiefly through the mucous membranes of the throat and nose. Few persons realize that the amount of air taken up by the system daily outweighs that of the solid food.

The changes which have taken place in the composition of the exhaled air are indicated by the following table:

Constituent	*Inhaled Air*	*Exhaled Air*
	—Volumes per cent—	
Nitrogen	78.35	78.85
Oxygen	20.77	16.
Carbon dioxide	0.04	4.35

Exhaled air is also saturated with water vapor and contains traces of ammonia and inorganic matter which vary with the diet, climate and occupation of the individual. Under normal conditions, if the blood is rich in the essential organic salts, especially iron, the lungs absorb through the medium of the red blood corpuscles twenty-four and one-half ounces of oxygen during twenty four hours, while they give off twenty-eight ounces of carbon dioxide in the same time. These amounts vary, of course, in different individuals in different occupations and under varied climatic conditions. Children need relatively more oxygen than do adults, as the tissue changes are more active during the growth of the organism.

During severe muscular exertion respiration is also increased in frequency and in depth, and the volume of air exchanged mav be from five to seven times greater than that required during a period of rest. Experiments have been made by German scientists showing the effect on oxygen consumption of walking on a level surface and when climbing. The following figures give the quantities of oxygen consumed during one minute, the subject being a man of 125 pounds weight.

Form of Exercise	*Oxygen Consumption*
Standing at rest	16 cubic inches
Walking on a level	48 cubic inches
Climbing	78 cubic inches

It appears that walking increases the consumption of oxygen three-fold, climbing nearly fivefold over that consumed when one is at rest. These facts illustrate the influence of muscular activity upon the exchange of matter in the body and the influence they exert in the purification of the system from waste matter. Regular exercise in the open air, during all seasons of the year, insuring a sufficient supply of oxygen, is one of the most important factors in the preservation of health and the prolongation of life.

CHAPTER IV

PURE WATER, A PRIME REQUISITE OF HEALTH

Water is one of the most characteristic substances of our planet. It may simultaneously appear solid, liquid and gaseous in form; it has been adapted as a unit of measure for the specific gravity of all other substances; it plays an important role in the circulation of the elements on the earth's surface. From oceans and lakes, fields and forests, a continuous stream of water is rising as vapor into the atmosphere, to be recondensed in cooler regions and precipitated as rain or snow. Three-fourths of these precipitations, of course, return directly to the ocean, the rest falling on land, collecting in rivers and lakes or else penetrating the earth, perhaps to be brought to the surface again as springs and wells. When water falls as rain to the earth, it absorbs carbon dioxide, ammonia and other soluble gases, if present, and washes the atmosphere free from dust-particles and impurities. This meteoric water (rain or snow), although nearly free from dissolved mineral substances, is therefore by no means pure, except at very high altitudes and above the line of perpetual ice and snow.

Good water should be clear, colorless, quite free from suspended matter, yet containing small quantities of carbon dioxide and atmospheric air to give it a pleasant, sparkling taste. In its chemical composition it ought to be as free as possible from organic matter and to contain not more than one-thousandth part of mineral matter or fifty grains per gallon. Unless the source of water is above suspicion, the water should be boiled, filtered or distilled. An addition of a small quantity of lime juice or lemon juice has also a purifying influence, on account of its large percentage of fruit acid.

Absolutely pure water can be obtained only by repeated distillations of fairly pure water in vessels constructed of silver. Distilled water, even when stored in porcelain or glass, quickly takes up small quantities of silicates, of which the containers are made. The purest water we can obtain in nature is the rain falling on a high mountain, or in the country after several hours of heavy precipitation.

Even rain water contains some minute solid particles, which are necessary for the condensation of the water vapor in the atmosphere, but the earthy matter of rain water is infinitesimal as compared with that of hard water. Bacteria are also present in rain water, which should be filtered if it is to be used for drinking purposes. Rain water is best stored in cement lined wells, as metal poisoning may occur from water stored in galvanized iron tanks. Decaying organic matter increases the solvent power of water for metals, thus corroding the containers and conveyance pipes. We hear of occasional cases of lead and zinc poisoning, resulting from water stored too long in galvanized tanks, which should never be used for this purpose.

Hard and Soft Water

All spring waters are more or less hard, the degree of hardness being generally determined by their capacity to dissolve soap. In soft water, such as rain water or distilled water, soap lathers immediately, while in hard water a considerable amount of soap is wasted before a lather is formed. This circumstance is caused by the calcium salts, carbonates and sulphate of lime, which unite with the fatty acids of the soap to produce new combinations. Only after these salts are chemically combined with the fatty acids can a satisfactory lather be made.

Calcium carbonate in spring water is formed by the presence of free carbonic acid gas (collected during its passage through the air as rain) which combines with the lime, taken up from the soil. Boiling the water breaks up the calcium carbonate into its component parts. The carbonic acid gas escapes into the air and the lime is precipitated; but unless calcium carbonate was the only mineral present, the water may still be hard, although less so than before. Chloride of calcium and sulphate of calcium cannot be removed by boiling; for isolating these substances there is no better remedy than that of distillation. If a still is used to purify the drinking water, such water, from which a part of the impurities have been altered, precipitated or removed by means of boiling or filtering, will not clog or coat the apparatus with lime as readily as do very hard waters.

The belief is without foundation that hard waters are beneficial because they furnish the necessary lime to the human system, and that soft water causes soft bones and premature decay of the teeth, or dissolves some of the necessary elements of the mucous membranes of the stomach and intestines. Distilled water will not attack any living tissue, as is often erroneously assumed. In fact, very hard waters often cause dyspepsia and constipation, which are relieved by the use of soft or distilled water.

Vegetables cooked in hard water are rendered hard and indigestible. This is especially the case with legumes, as the sulphate of calcium in water, when boiled, forms hard, indigestible compounds with the legumin, causing flatulency. There is no doubt that the use of distilled water tends to prolong life as it prevents to a large extent the ossification of the arteries and it lessens the work of the kidneys.

Water is necessary to all forms of vegetable and animal life, even the lowest types. The change of matter into human energy is dependent upon the presence of water in the tissues. No vital action is possible without it. It constitutes nearly two-thirds of the human body.

The presence of water is essential in the processes of digestion and absorption, as a solvent for foods. It is likewise necessary for dissolving the various substances which have to be removed from the body through the excretory organs. More than one-half of the amount of water taken into the system is again discharged through the kidneys, about one-quarter through the skin, seventeen per cent through the lungs and four per cent through the intestines. Thus we are constantly losing water in various ways. The air we exhale is saturated with moisture and the skin is daily giving off from one to two pints of water in the form of invisible perspiration, or in the form of sweat during strenuous exercise.

Our Daily Requirements of Water

The amount of water actually needed by the body depends on various circumstances, principally on climate and occupation. The greater the functional activity of the organism, the greater the need for fluid. This need is indicated by thirst which is best satisfied by pure water, but the larger part of the water necessary for the physiological functions of the system may be derived from our food, if judiciously selected. Thus fruits contain a very large percentage of water, from 80 to 90 per cent, so that people partaking freely of fresh fruits and vegetables need little or no water in addition to that supplied by their food. *Furthermore, in nature's products, we get the water in the purest form, distilled in her own laboratory,* and this is undoubtedly the best and most hygienic way in which water may be taken. Besides, in fruits and vegetables, the water is in an organic combination with other elements and in this state it has the most beneficial action upon our system. A person living largely upon these foods has very little desire for any liquid. It is only the excessive consumption of meat and of other highly seasoned foods which create an abnormal thirst. Certain animals, such as hares, and rabbits, which feed on grasses and herbs containing about 85% of water, never drink so long as they can find their natural food. Mother's milk contains about 87% of water; juicy fruits and succulent vegetables also possess almost the same fluidic content. A person who consumes about four pounds of fresh fruit daily absorbs in addition to about eight ounces of solid food, at least three pints of water of unsurpassed quality.

As already stated, in case of a high protein diet more water is necessary than is required on a diet consisting largely of foods in which fats and carbohydrates predominate. This is because the waste products of the former need a larger amount of water for their solution and excretion. However, we should not maintain that by copious water drinking we are able to flush the system like a sewer. This is a mistaken view coming from a lack of understanding of the physiological function of the system. Purification of the human organism is an electro-chemical process of the living cells. The waste products like those of uric acid, sulphuric acid, carbonic acid, etc., must be first combined with some of the alkaline elements, principally sodium, before they can be taken up by the blood stream and excreted.

As already pointed out, the best way to regulate the water supply of the system is to adopt a simple and frugal diet, containing a liberal supply of salad plants and fresh fruits, and free from spices and condiments. Thus the desire for liquids will be greatly appeased and, whenever thirst does occur, it will be a natural one which can be best quenched with pure and soft water in moderate quantity.

If liquids for which there is no physiological need are habitually taken into the system it is certainly not in accordance with the laws of hygiene. No strict rules in regard to the quantity of water can be made, except that drinking during meals should be avoided, or at least reduced to the minimum. A meal of fresh fruit satisfies thirst, especially during warm weather. Ice water should never be taken, and the temperature of drinking water should never be much below that of 50 degrees Fahrenheit. When the use of hot water is required internally, the temperature should be between 110 and 120 degrees Fahrenheit.

CHAPTER V

EXERCISE AND REST, A VITAL NECESSITY

Bodily exercise is nature's method of accelerating the circulation of the blood, of forcing from the system clogging waste and of strengthening the muscles. Exercise is quite as important as is diet, for without exercise we cannot properly digest our food, no matter how wholesome it is. Today the automobile, while a great time saver, is depriving us of an abundance of exercise, especially of the lower extremities. If you would take your car to some interesting place, then devote some time to brisk walk, mountain climbing, swimming or rowing you would increase your physical endurance. Regular daily gymnastics in the open air should be taken by all who live a sedentary indoor life.

The physiological effects of exercise upon the different bodily organs make physical culture a hygienic necessity. Moderate exercise increases the size of the muscles, renders them harder and less sensitive to injury, and through the agency of the nervous system they become trained to a readier performance of movement of every kind. The beneficial changes in muscle-fibre resulting from exercise are due to the increased blood supply which is called forth by muscular contraction, resulting in increased nutrition and growth. Excessive exercise of any set of muscles induces hypertrophy, and this may eventually result in stiffness and in lessened capacity for activity.

The chemical reaction of muscle is changed to acid during exercise. The venous blood contains more carbonic acid than that occuring under ordinary exertion, demonstrating that active molecular changes are going on, stimulated by exercise. Scientific experiments have shown that in a state of bodily rest, the absorption of oxygen in twelve hours amounted to 709 grams (about 25 oz.); during work the amount reached 945 grams (about 34 oz.). For the same period the elimination of carbonic acid was, during rest, 911 grams (32½ oz.); during work 1284 grams (46 oz.). In other words the absorption of oxygen and the elimination of carbonic acid was about one-third more during work than that exchanged during rest.

How to Increase Our Endurance

According to Professor A. V. Hill, an English physiologist, the direct cause of the fatigue resulting from muscular effort is the accumulation of lactic acid, the source of which is glycogen. The body stores up carbohydrates in the form of glycogen or liver starch, which is used up during muscular activity. The excessive accumulation of lactic acid in the blood is the result of an insufficient intake of oxygen by the system. If the iron and sodium contents of the blood are below normal, due to faulty diet, both the absorption of oxygen and the discharge of carbonic acid are diminished, lactic acid accumulates in the muscles; the latter subsequently stiffen and fail to function—the sign of fatigue.

It is therefore of great importance for athletes and for those who are subjected to muscular strain, to maintain a high degree of alkalinity of the blood by avoiding as much as possible highly acid-forming foods (meat, eggs, legumes, etc.), and by consuming an adequate supply of fruits and green-leaf vegetables. When proper attention is paid to diet, fatigue, especially during strenuous exercise, is retarded, while endurance is increased. The Japanese, Chinese, and some of the Hindu tribes living in the Himalaya mountains, who subsist on frugal diet and hardly eat any meat, possess a most remarkable physical stamina. These facts are worthy of careful attention, not only by athletes, but by all who want to derive much benefit from their regular exercise.

Benefits Derived from Regular Exercise

The involuntary muscles of the body, as for example those in the stomach and the intestinal canal, are strengthened by the exercise of their fibres equally as much as are the voluntary or external muscles; and the solid or muscular structures of the body, such as the heart and the uterus, are improved in functional activity by the physiological process initiated by the voluntary muscles.

Difficult and painful menstruation is often relieved by general systematic exercise and an alkaline diet, without the need for recourse to any other measures. The normal growth and development of the bones of the body are evidently influenced by that of systematic exercise. The functional improvement of the nervous mechanism represented by any movement, involuntary or voluntary, is the most important effect of muscular exertion.

As the circulation of the blood is accelerated by exercise, a larger quantity of air is required to areate the blood. The lungs, therefore, act more quickly, more air is inhaled and a larger amount of carbonic acid is exhaled. Ordinarily, a man inhales about 500 cubic inches of air per minute. By walking about 4 miles per hour he draws in about 2500 cubic inches per minute, or five times more than that absorbed when sitting in his automobile.

Walking is one of the most simple and valuable of the exercises that are taken in the open air. Taken at a good swinging pace in comfortable attire, not obstructing the free movements of the muscles, it is most beneficial for the normal functions of the heart and lungs, especially developing the lower limbs, and the spinal muscles which keep the body erect. Children and others should be taught to walk erect, to hold the chest out, and to cultivate an easy gait; this may be assisted by proper gymnastic training. Walking is especially beneficial to those who are subjected to the routine of office or shop work every day.

One of the finest exercises is swimming. It should be practiced as much as possible out-of-doors during the summer and indoors during cool or cold weather. Nearly all cities are now provided with indoor swimming tanks, which make possible this wholesome exercise during all seasons of the year. Swimming is particularly desirable for children, because of the influence it exerts in developing the chest and back, as well as in giving symmetrical exercise to the body. Remember "the child is father to the man." The foundation of a strong and healthy body is laid during childhood and before birth. Children should be given every opportunity to grow into healthy and strong men and women by permitting them to take adequate exercise in the open air as often as possible.

Sleep, an Alkalinizer

Adequate rest is necessary to protect the alkalinity of the blood, because waste matter of the body is mostly eliminated during rest and sleep, and the body is constantly being alkalinized during this period. It is therefore absolutely essential that we give ourselves a sufficient amount of rest and sleep, especially after a time of strenuous activity.

The ever active growing child requires more sleep than does the adult. The growing child is, moreover, less tolerant of an acid condition of the body than is the adult. Hence he needs a greater amount of rest and sleep, and a higher percentage of foods which produce an alkaline reaction in the body. It is during the night, when we are at rest, that the lungs redouble their efforts to inhale the life-giving oxygen to recharge the human dynamo for another day of useful activity. We should therefore always sleep near open windows or at least in well ventilated rooms.

CHAPTER VI

THE INFLUENCE OF MIND ON HEALTH

The brain and nervous system represents the highest physical development of the body. The brain directs the voluntary muscles in the performance of mechanical work, also the organs of speech and it controls numerous other voluntary and commonly performed actions. But it is now more and more realized by profound students that our mental attitude can directly influence the numerous complicated and delicate functions of the body which are involved in the maintenance of health and the prevention of disease. In fact the brain is merely the organ of the mind which is constantly receiving reports from various parts of the physical body. The mind is able to influence the health and action of the entire body through the nervous regulation and control of the cellular and glandular secretions.

Disease is now generally recognized to be either a derangement of the functions of the cell, or a degeneration of the substance of the cell, aggravated by faulty foods. Our health is entirely dependent upon the health of one and all of the many millions of cells that compose the physical body. But we cannot deny that the mind is able to influence and more or less control the entire nutrition and metabolism of the body. By regulating and modifying the cellular and glandular secretions of the entire body, the mind by means of the nervous system, controls the nutrition, growth and life history of all the body cells.

It has been proved time and again that joyful emotions increase the assimilative powers of the body; while fear retards, delays and even temporarily inhibits the process of assimilation, even if we partake of the best of foods.

The Detrimental Effects of Fear and Worry

The greatest obstacles to nature's healing efforts are fear and worry. To the extent which the patient is impressed with the constant dread of germs and infection—instead of awakening his faith in the ever active, innate natural healing forces—his ultimate recovery will be retarded. Fear and worry always interfere with the rhythm of all the vital functions of the organism, lessening the power of resistance. In striking contrast, joyful emotions heighten the activity of all the organs and glands of the body. Under the influence of joy the small arteries and capillaries dilate and every organ receives an increased and more active blood supply.

Through the influence of joy upon the muscular system there is not only an increased disposition of activity, but an increased capacity for effort and endurance. The heart beats stronger, the brain thinks clearer, breathing is deeper, digestion more active, the eyes brighter, the cheeks glow, the whole body rejoices and prospers under the influence of a peaceful, contented mental state.

CHAPTER VII

FOOD, NATURAL AND ARTIFICIAL

The battle for supremacy, which is now going on in all fields of human endeavor, has more than ever brought the question to the front: "How shall we live to develop the greatest energy and perseverance mentally and physically and at the same time strenghen our resistance against fatigue and disease?" The interest in solving this problem is growing deeper every year, and there is no doubt that man can wonderfully increase his capacity for work, with body and mind, by proper selection of his food according to the principles of physiology and bio-chemistry (chemistry of life).

The transmutation of air, food and drink into blood and tissues, and thence into muscular and mental energy, is of course a biological process, which is common to all animals. But it is given to the intellect of man to select understandingly from the quality of his food a sufficiency of those elements which are essential to the maintenance of health and efficiency. Nevertheless, it is only in the animal world that health is the normal condition because wild animals, moved by natural impulse, not by faulty reasoning, live in a natural environment. With civilized mankind we find the condition almost reversed; absolute health is exceptional, while the majority of people are suffering from more or less severe physical ailments, or at least show physical and mental lassitude.

In every civilized country the cost of sickness and lowered mental and physical efficiency runs into billions of dollars every year. It is therefore not too much to assert that the solution of many social and economic problems of today would be greatly helped if attention were given to the question of food and rational nutrition.

Natural Foods Are the Best

We are living in an age of commercialism where the quick accumulation of material wealth seems to dominate civilized man, frequently at the cost of his physical and mental welfare. Despite the ever increasing number of schools and colleges, he remains lamentably ignorant of the most important and fundamental factors on which health and happiness depend. In fact, in few fields of study and observation have human need been more inadequately met than in that of the chemistry of foods and nutrition as related to our physical and mental well being. Few people understand the true meaning of natural foods, for they have been fed from childhood upon unnatural, artificially prepared foods, which are detrimental to the normal function of the digestive organs and gradually impair our health. Civilized man is manufacturing and eating many substances that slowly but surely lead to degeneration, disease and premature death.

As a result of our great industrial development, millions of people, especially those living in the larger cities, are far away from the source of their food supply and many articles of food and food preparations reach the consumer in an impoverished and adulterated condition. Even farmers ship their natural whole grain to the flour mills; they then turn over to the canneries their fruits and vegetables, and buy back at fancy prices devitalized cereal products, pickled, canned and preserved foods. There is no doubt that many indispositions and diseases are caused by faulty and inadequate nutrition, and that the restoration and preservation of health can be augmented by the judicious use of such foods as are produced under ideal conditions and remain is as nearly a natural state as possible when they are consumed.

The growth and ripening of foods in field, orchard and garden in their endless varieties and the processes of digestion and assimilation which take place in the living organism have not the same relationship as that of the test tube of the chemical laboratory. The organic world, the plant and animal kingdom, is dependent on the chemical combinations of the elements, the soil, water and air, elaborated by the sunlight and that mysterious life-giving force which is contained in the protoplasm of every germ.

The Wonderful Chemistry of the Living Body

The human body is composed of a number of elements, all of which are important in the various physiological functions of the organism. Our food should not only contain the elements for the renewal of the tissues, the production of heat and energy, for the elaboration of the digestive juices for the secretions of the ductless glands, but also a surplus of the alkaline elements which neutralize the poisons constantly arising from processes of oxidation in the cells. All the material manifestations of life and growth are very closely interwoven with the chemical actions and reactions of these elements; hence the problem of healthy and adequate nutrition of the body can never be solved without paying careful attention to the physiological functions of the organic salts.

The mechanical part of food absorption by the body may be explained by the laws of diffusion and osmosis. But the wall of the intestine does not behave like a dead membrane. Every epithelial cell is in itself an organism, a living being.

The activity of the glands and the processes of secretion show the same wonderful power of selection, of picking out certain constituents of the blood, of altering them by the processes of synthesis and decomposition, of sending them into the ducts of the glands, and others back into the blood and lymph. The epithelial cells of the mammary glands collect from normal blood all the substances in the right proportion for the production of mother's milk, which has an entirely different composition from that present in the blood. We can not imitate these subtle processes of nature; thus the dream of some enterprising chemists to produce artifically foodstuffs that sustain life and growth may never be realized.

The Failure of Synthetic Foods

For life and health and for the prevention of bodily disorders no laboratory concoction can equal the indispensable products of organic nature. No substances other than the highly organized products of nature are biologically appropriate or fit for the maintenance of the life of bodily cells and nothing else can safely be introduced into the human organism. Although the chemist is able to build up artificially a series of more or less complex organic compounds, his experiments do not represent the synthetic processes of the living cell. All of the so-called organic substances coming from the laboratory are produced by the application of forces and agents which can never play a part in the vital processes; such as extreme pressure, high temperature, strong galvanic currents, etc., agencies which would be immediately fatal to the living cell.

To take an extreme case, how can a chemist imitate an apple? No amount of analysis and subsequent synthesis will enable him to do so, for though he were to succeed in reproducing the elements in their due proportions, and even some of their chemical combinations, still there is a bloom of life about the fruit that will defy his efforts.

Henry Ford, the mechanical wizard, was recently quoted in a newspaper item as follows:

> "Machine processes can manufacture milk more efficiently than the crude system used by the cow. It is a simple matter to take the same cereals that cows eat and make them into milk that is superior to the natural article and free from tuberculosis germs. Our laboratories have demonstrated that fact."

Nothing could be farther from the truth. Aside from the facts that the cow needs an ample supply of green fodder for the production of good milk, and that the chemical composition of cereals is entirely different from that of the milk of any animals, milk is not an essential factor in the nutrition of mammals including man,—that is after they have been weaned. The laboratory processes of making milk from cereals are very crude indeed as compared with the wonderful synthetic work performed by the living cells of the mammary glands, in producing a vital fluid that is physiologically and biologically adapted to the needs of the newborn in the various stages of growth during the nursing period.

One of the scientific delusions that break into print every little while is that in the future man will go to the drug store for his food, as he has gone, and as countless deluded people still go, for their bane. The following dispatch appeared in the daily newspapers several years ago:

> "A future day when a large part of the world's food supply will be artificially produced, emancipating man from absolute dependence on the soil," was depicted in an address before the American Chemical Society, in convention here, today by Dr. Carl Alsberg, director of the Food Research Bureau of Leland Stanford University. "There is every reason to believe," Dr. Alsberg declared, "that the three basic groups of foodstuffs—carbohydrates, fats, and the amino-acids—can and shortly will be producible by artificial means."
>
> "The most promising source of energy for mankind to turn to in the 'day of artificial food production'," Dr. Alsberg said, "is solar radiation. By a mechanical process of storing up the heat units of the sun," he declared, "the present 'inefficiency of agriculture, due to its 'waste of energy,' would be largely supplanted by the efficiency of a chemical process."

Nature's Inimitable Laboratory

There are in nature's organic products subtle qualities which are not susceptible to chemical analysis, and these are too volatile to survive the laboratory processes of extraction and condensation. The ingredients revealed by the material analyses of foods are believed to be the essential constituents. Here, too, it is probable that these ingredients are not the most valuable, but only the coarser part. It has been proved that every living cell is a storage battery of organic electricity whose subtle power of maintaining the life processes is easily diminished or often entirely dissipated through prolonged boiling or other deleterious influences. The principal function of food is not simply to be digested and oxidized in the tissue cells, as present day physiology assumes, but to supply electrical "ions." We may safely say that the ultimate source of animal heat and nerve force which keeps up the vigorous health of all vital organs is electricity, which is chiefly stored up in the sun-ripened fruits, nuts, cereals, vegetables, in their natural state.

The many manufactured and artifically compounded foods that have been made available and are constantly produced as wonderful remedies, would soon be discredited as failures if any number of people would attempt to live on them exclusively for a given period. The fact cannot be emphasized too much that food that builds and perpetuates the human race must be compounded in nature's great laboratory, planned by the cosmic intelligence; the process must be evolutionary, and time is not one of the least of the elements in the process. Many millions of years had to pass before man could make his appearance on this planet, and before proper food for his life and propagation could be evolved.

Solar and Chemical Energy

Few people realize the titanic forces which were instrumental in the evolution of the organic world, and which are progressively ever active. The sunlight potential, which performs the work of energy and is stored up in the plant, corresponds to that attained at a temperature of 10,000 degrees Fahrenheit. The importance of this measurement of the light potential is readily apparent in the relation of chemical energy and sunlight energy, as it is stored up in the products of the soil. The driving force of life is the transformed energy of the sunlight. The primary conversion of certain rays of the sun and of their use in making the complex substances of protoplasm takes place in the green leaves of the plant. The green pigment of chlorophyll seems to be the starting point of organized vegetative life. Chlorophyll itself is the result of uncounted millions of years of evolution from jelly-like substances, emanating and evolved from the primeval sea millions of years ago. Some plants, which have no chlorophyll or leaf-green, live like leaches on the products of other species, which furnish this wonderful material.

Out of the sunlight originates the chemical energy with which the wisdom of life fulfills its purposes and plans. We cannot nourish ourselves with proximate principles, such as protein, fat, carbohydrates, minerals and vitamins, artifically combined. There never will be a condensed food, prepared and pressed into tablets, which will meet all nutritional requirements of the complex human organism.

We can never expect to explain fully the processes of life by the laws of physics and chemistry alone. The more thoroughly and conscientiously we endeavor to study biological problems, the more are we convinced that even those processes which we have already regarded as explicable by chemical and physical laws, are in reality, infinitely more complex, and at present defy anv attempt at a mechanical explanation. Future generations may overcome the stupendous difficulties which at present beset physiological and biological investigations, and may come nearer to solving the mysteries of life which now puzzle the minds of the profoundest students of nature.

CHAPTER VIII

THE CONSTITUENTS OF FOOD

Considered in the Light of Modern Biology

While there are more than a thousand food-products, their constituents or proximate principles are always about the same, although they are found in varying proportions. We shall here briefly enumerate these constituents and deal with them more explicitly in the following pages.

Water, composed of hydrogen and oxygen, is contained in varying percentages in all natural foods. It is indispensable as a solvent in all the physiological functions of the body and of every form of life.

Nitrogenous compounds, chiefly found in the form of *protein,* are composed of carbon, oxygen, hydrogen and sulphur. They rebuild the wear and tear of the tissues and furnish also some potential energy when there is more supplied than that needed for functional purposes. The protoplasm or both the plant and animal cell is composed mainly of protein. Protein, again exists in various forms, such as the *albumen* of eggs, the *casein* of milk, the *gluten* of cereals, the *legumin* of pulses, etc. Similar to protein in chemical composition are the *gelatins* which, however, do not assist in repairing the waste of the tissues, but serve as a source of heat and energy. About fifty different proteins have been sufficiently isolated and studied. Their nitrogen contents range from 15.50 per cent in egg albumen to about 18 per cent in gluten found in wheat and other cereals. The *amino-acids* are nitrogenous compounds of simpler structure than are the proteins. Seventeen different kinds have been determined so far. In the construction of the protein molecules of plants, nitrogen is absorbed from the soil in soluble forms, as compounds of nitrates and ammonium salts, which are converted first into amino-acids and then into protein. The reverse takes place in the animal body, where the protein molecule is again broken up into simpler compounds like amino acids and finally into ammonia, urea, uric acid. etc., which in the open air undergo oxidation and re-conversion into nitrates and ammonium salts, ready to be taken up again by the plant.

Non-nitrogenous compounds. These exist in the form of *carbohydrates and fats,* and are always made up of the same three elements: carbon, hydrogen. oxygen.

The carbohydrates are chiefly products of the vegetable kingdom, such as sugars, starches, cellulose, gums, pectins and dextrins. In the milk of mammals, however, we find a considerable amount of carbohydrates in the form of milk sugar. Carbohydrates are not directly required, like protein, to build up or repair the cells of the body, but they are readily oxidized by the inhaled air into carbon dioxide and water, furnishing heat and energy to the system with the greatest vital economy.

Fats are found mainly in the seeds of plants and to some extent in the leaves. skins and fruits; they are also found in most of the animal food products. Fats are deficient in oxygen and rich in carbon and hydrogen. Consequently their heat-equivalent is much greater than that of the carbohydrates. The latter yield 1,820 calories per pound, the former more than twice as much or 4,040 calories.

The fats and the carbohydrates may replace each other, but only within certain limits. They do not appear to play exactly the same part, although composed of the same elements. The fact that fat is contained in the milk of all mammals, in the eggs and in all seeds of plants, seems to demonstrate that it is an indispensable food constituent. It is further proved by the instinctive desire for the addition of fat to a diet, however abundant in carbohydrates it may be, and the desire, on the other hand, for the addition of carbohydrates to the richest fat diet.

To the non-nitrogenous compounds also belong the *organic acids* of the vegetable kingdom, such as tartaric acid, citric acid, and malic acid, which are likewise oxidized into carbon dioxide and water, supplying heat and energy to the system.

While carbohydrates and fats cannot replace protein, a deficiency of nitrogen is made good, to a limited extent, by the protective agency of the other food stuffs which offer themselves for all the offices except the final one of tissue building. The fat of all foods is very completely absorbed, far more so than is the protein. The same is true of all carbohydrates, with the single exception of cellulose.

The *vitamins,* several of which have been discovered so far, whose chemical composition is now definitely known, are present in varying quantities in all natural foods. They are intimately connected with the processes of life and growth, but they can be active only when all the body-building elements are present in the right quantities and proportions.

The *organic salts or mineral elements* play the most important part in our nutrition. In articles on foods and tables of food-contents, they generally figure under the collective names of mineral matter, ash or inorganic foodstuffs, without any attention being paid to their elementary composition. Their study has been woefully neglected by the majority of physiologists who have treated them as unimportant substances. We are constantly confronted with such statements as these: "The part which each of the mineral elements plays in animal nutrition is not well understood," or that "with the ordinary mixed diet the body demands for mineral matter may be met." *but as long as the importance of the organic salts in our system is not recognized and understood, just so long will there exist such deplorable guesswork, both with regard to diagnosis and the treatment of diseases.***

To enjoy perfect health and immunity from disease, our blood must contain all the necessary elements in their wonderful organic combinations; because it is the blood which carries them to the different parts of the body, nourishing and cleansing the tissues, creating animal heat, magnetism and electricity.

** Fortunately great advances are being made today.

In recapitulating the different constituents of food, we may divide them into three classes:

(1) Those which replace the worn-out tissue elements of the body and at the same time supply heat and energy, such as proteins, and fats;

(2) Those which supply heat and energy only, such as carbohydrates, gelatins and the inhaled oxygen of the air;

(3) Those which repair only the worn-out tissues, such as water and organic salts, the latter through their electro-magnetic properties being most essential in all the vital functions of the organism. The organic salts are of as great importance to the animal and human organism as are the proteins, fats and carbohydrates combined.

As previously mentioned, no proximate food-principle alone is able to sustain vital force in the animal organism, and the above division is merely provisional. Fats may be placed in the first as well as in the second class, while gelatins and carbohydrates may indirectly assist in the building up of cells, by protecting the tissues from decomposition and oxidation.

Protein, Only a Small Amount Required If the Diet Is Rich in Alkaline Elements

While proteins in the different forms are necessary for our nutrition, the required amount for our daily needs has been greatly over-estimated. The craving for concentrated protein foods like that of meat is one of man's acquired habits and has led to many diseased conditions. Since our muscular tissues consist chiefly of protein, the early students of physiology supposed that this constituent was the source of muscular energy. In fact it has been one of the physiological dogmas of the past that the tissues and organs of the body, or rather their constituent cells, must be supplied with protein for all their functions whenever it was available. The remarkable fact that the output of nitrogen is equivalent to the intake of protein; that the body cannot store up nitrogen to any considerable extent, has been mistaken as conclusive evidence that the organism prefers to use protein for most of its requirements.

Today we know that in muscular work under rational nutrition the excretion of nitrogen is increased only to a very slight degree, that the absorption of oxygen and the excretion of carbonic acid is notably increased; that, therefore, muscular energy is mainly derived from non-nitrogenous substances, like sugar and starch, as they exist in natural foods. The oxidation of the elements of food usually takes place in the active tissues, but, according to our present knowledge of matter, it does not seem to occur at the expense of protein in living cells. In other words, it is not the protein incorporated in the cells that undergoes change, but the protein circulating in and about the internal meshes of the cells and tissues, the living cell being the active agent in controlling the process. Only the carbon contained in protein is utilized in the production of heat and energy, while the system has to excrete the surplus of nitrogen, overtaxing liver and kidneys.

The fuel value of protein, containing as it does from fifty per cent to fifty-five per cent of carbon, is not greater than that of an equal amount of sugar or starch, and less than half of that of fats. A number of careful experiments by German scientists demonstrated that the amount of protein used could safely be reduced to 40 grams (1½ ounces), or to about one-third of the usual amount of 120 grams (4½ ounces). But the old standards of Liebig and Voit had been so firmly established in the minds of the medical profession, that these experiments merely excited comment without changing to any extent the prevalent belief of the necessity of large amounts of protein to maintain health and strength.

Professor Jaffa's Experiments

In the United States extended experiments have been made by Professor Jaffa of the University of California at Berkeley, and Dr. Russel H. Chittenden of Yale University at New Haven, Connecticut. Professor Jaffa's report of investigations made among a number of fruitarians, contains an interesting account of a dietary study of a family of fruitarians consisting of two women and three children. They all had been fruitarians from five to seven years, their diet consisting chiefly of fruits and nuts, with the addition of celery, honey, olive oil, and occasionally a small amount of prepared cereal foods.

On this frugal diet, which consisted chiefly of uncooked foods, excluding all animal foods and legumes, this family with three growing children had lived in good health all these years. All the members of the family were put under observation for about three weeks. The food consumed was carefully weighed and the chemical composition determined. The average amount of food consumed per day was: 33 grams (1-1/5 ounces) of protein, 59 grams (2 ounces) of fat, 150 grams (7-1/3 ounces) of carbohydrates, with a total of about 11 ounces of solid food (about 1500 calories).

While the menus outlined by Dr. Chittenden are better than are those of the average American dietary still they leave room for improvement. If the alkaline elements are not furnished in the right proportion the cells of the body are broken down, in order to make up for the deficiency in our diet. Thus the mineral reserves of our body are depleted, thereby lowering our powers of resistance. Nature's best eliminators of waste poison are the alkaline elements, especially sodium, calcium and iron, liberally supplied in the form of fruits and green-leaf vegetables. Health and efficiency can be maintained on a diet furnishing no more than an ounce, or two ounces of protein at the utmost even under severe muscular and mental exertion.

The Advantages of a Low Protein Diet

Attention should be called here to the painstaking investigations of Dr. M. Hindhede of Copenhagen, Denmark, published in his book "Protein and

Nutrition," and also to the experiments of Dr. C. Roese, of Erfurt, Germany, which were explained in his brochure, "Over Consumption of Protein and Under Consumption of Basic Elements." All these careful investigations prove beyond doubt that the normal body weight can be maintained and our health and endurance increased on an alkaline diet furnishing even less than two ounces of protein per day. As has been repeatedly emphasized, it is the presence of a sufficient amount of alkaline elements in our blood which protects the protein molecule of the tissues against premature cleavage and disintegration.

It is evident that a diet high in protein and in other acid-forming foods means the consumpton of heavy meals, an excess of waste products, retarded elimination, and of susceptibility to disease. A diet low in protein but rich in alkaline elements means smaller quantities of food, fewer waste products, quick elimination, together with excellent physical and mental health and endurance.

The low protein requirement of man's normal diet are distinctly proved by the changes which occur in mother's milk at the different stages of the child's development. Under normal conditions the mammary glands of the mother supply less protein as the infant grows older, so that after six months the percentage of protein in mother's milk has decreased from 2.38 per cent to 1.07 per cent.

These are certainly excellent proofs that our daily requirement of protein is much smaller than that which has been so far assumed. The necessary amount of from one to about two ounces per day for the adult man can easily be supplied by a judicious selection of the products of the vegetable kingdom. The excessive consumption of meat, especially in the United States, causes an enormous amount of loss both from the standpoint of health and economy.

Carbohydrates (Sugars, Starches, Etc.)

Carbohydrates comprise a number of chemically related substances: the sugars of different kinds; the various forms of starch in its normal condition, as well as those in soluble form, such as dextrins, etc.; the gums, pectins, or jelly-like bodies; and finally fiber and cellulose. They contain on an average 44 per cent carbon, 6 per cent hydrogen, 50 percent oxygen.

They are subdivided according to their chemical composition into three distinct groups:

1. *Monosaccharides* comprising *grape sugar* (dextrose or glucose); *fruit sugar* (fructose or levulose), and *galactose* (derived from milk sugar.)

2. *Disaccharides* comprising *sucrose* (saccharose or cane sugar) found often combined with dextrose and fructose in the juice of many fruits and vegetables; *maltose* (malt-sugar) formed from starch by enzymic action, and *lactose* (milk sugar) found in the milk of all mammals.

3. *Polysaccharides.* They include *starch,* in which form nature stores most

of the carbohydrates in the vegetable kingdom; *glycogen,* which is stored as reserve carbohydrate prncipally in the liver and muscular tissues of the animals; *dextrins,* which are formed from starch by diastase, acid or heat; *cellulose,* principally found in wood and in the cell walls of plants; *galactans,* which occur in seeds of legumes and cereals, in some of the algae and lichens, and the *pectins* or jelly-like bodies. To this group also belong the *pentosans,* which generally are found in the fibrous tissues and gummy exudations of plants, but not in the starchy and succulent parts.

By the chemical addition of a certain amount of water the second and third groups can be converted into substances of the first. This process is called inversion and may be produced in a number of ways.

Natural Sugars, Superior to Refined Sugar

Grape-sugar and fruit-sugar exist together in most of the sweet fruits and honey, and although they have the same chemical composition, they are not identical bodies. This is accounted for by their peculiar molecular structure, the same number of atoms being arranged in a different way.

Cane sugar (sucrose) is two and one-half times sweeter than is grape-sugar. It exists in many vegetable juices. It is found in the stems and roots of all the grasses, especially in the sugar cane and sorghum; in succulent roots, such as the carrot, turnip, red beet, sweet potato and sugar beet; in the sap of trees such as the date palm and sugar maple; also to a small extent in all sweet fruits, and in the nectar of flowers. The commercial manufacture of refined sugar beets and sugar cane has developed from crude beginnings. In olden times sugar was quite an expensive luxury, mostly imported from the Orient. In the latter part of the nineteenth century the manufacture of refined sugar from sugar cane and sugar beets developed to such an extent, both in America and Europe, that it is now one of the great staples of commerce.

Cane sugar cannot be utilized directly in the body. By the action of a ferment in the intestine known as *invertin* it is converted into mono-saccharides, that is, changed into levulose and glucose which are ready for immediate absorption and use in the system. The change of cane sugar in solution into dextrose and levulose can also be brought about to some extent by the action of heat and diluted acids, as in cooking acid fruits with cane sugar.

Maltose, belonging to the same group of disaccharides, is produced in sprouting grains by a digestive process which converts the starch into sugar. The unorganized ferment, or enzyme, which accomplishes this change is known as *diastase.* A similar ferment is able to convert raw starch into maltose, which may be absorbed without undergoing change in the intestine.

It should be borne in mind, however, that the various forms of sugar, such as those found in their natural state in fruits, stems and in roots, are organized by nature during the process of growth, and are intimately associated with other nourishing constituents. Sugars in the form of natural food products are infinitely better than are the manufactured refined sweets of commerce, which are chemically isolated food principles and can never fully supply the needs of the body.

Why Refined Sugar Is Injurious

The reason for the injurious effects of manufactured refined cane sugar is that it is artificially extracted and separated from those organic combinations which are necessary for the building up of tissues and bones, for the proper functioning of the nervous system and the purification of the blood. Without a constant renewal of the elements of iron and sodium, the blood cannot take up sufficient oxygen and the products of combustion cannot be neutralized and eliminated. The blood stream is overloaded with waste products, causing sluggishness and general drowsiness, the symptoms of carbonic acid poisoning.

The extensive use of artificial sweets, especially in connection with starchy foods is responsible for a large number of diseases of the digestive organs. The liver and kidneys are severely affected by the increased formation of toxic substances, and the accumulation of acids in the blood, cause a catarrhal condition of all the mucous membranes. Not enough can be said in warning against the prevalent and extensive use of refined sugar in the various forms of pastry and confectionery. That the general public is not aware of the injurious effects of refined sweets, seems to be indicated by the rapid increase in the manufacture and consumption of sugar.

Figures gathered by the Bureau of Statistics show that the average American consumes about 110 pounds of sugar every year, and that Uncle Sam's sugar bill averages over two million dollars a day. The total consumption of sugar in the United States amounts to about thirteen billion pounds. Calculating this enormous total at the average retail price of 5 cents per pound, we get a total of $650,000,000 as its cost to the consumers.

Whatever interest these figures may possess from a commercial standpoint, considered from a hygienic point of view, they are deplorable. Indeed, the use of artificial sweets is one of the most pernicious customs of the day, causing defective development of the skeleton of the infantile body, and in later years a morbid softening of the bones, making dentistry one of the most lucrative professions in this country.

Taste for Sweets is Natural

The taste for sweets is natural, and indicates a physiological demand. This demand, however, can be met only by the natural sugars existing principally in sweet fruits. The nutritious and fattening qualities of the whole sugar cane, for instance, are sufficiently shown on every sugar estate. With their free use of the cane, the negroes of the West Indies and every animal about the plantation at the time of harvest show conclusively the wholesome and nutritious properties of the cane juice. This is but another illustration of the fact that we cannot improve on nature; for in the ripened cane, sugar is organized with other constituents, making it a more balanced food.

Some of the sugar that is not immediately needed in the system is manufactured by the liver into glycogen and is stored up in that organ and in the muscles for future use in the performance of muscular work. The habitual indulgence in sugar in the concentrated form, such as syrups, refined sugar candies, preserves, etc., causes fatty degeneration of the organs of the body. This condition is known to be the foundation of such disorders as diabetes, fatty heart and abnormal conditions of the liver, kidneys, muscles and bones. Again, sugar in great excess of that which the liver can take care of causes fermentation in the alimentary canal, producing alcohol, carbonic acid and acetic acid. Like all other acquired tastes, the sugar eating habit is hard to give up, but numerous tests have shown that when the habit is once broken, the natural taste of food appears more pleasant than when it is disguised by the presence of manufactured refined sugar.

Milk sugar, or lactose, is similar in chemical composition to that of cane sugar, but is not nearly so sweet. It is a constituent of the milk of all mammals in various percentages, ranging from two to eight per cent. Barring dextrose, it is the most digestible sugar for infants. When milk is exposed to the air, the milk sugar undergoes decomposition whereby lactic acid is formed and the milk becomes sour. In fermentation one molecule of milk sugar takes up one of water and splits into four of lactic acid.

Starch — Nature's Storehouse of Carbohydrates

Starch, next to water, is the substance most abundant in the average diet of man, largely due to the circumstance that the foods which contain it can be produced cheaply. In nature starches are never found in their proximate form —they are always intimately connected with other food-elements of the protoplasmic cell.

Starch is the form in which nature stores up the carbohydrates in seeds and roots for future use. If she should store away sugar instead of starch it would be dissolved by the first rainstorm, and every rain would spoil the seed; but raw starch is insoluble and at the same time unfermentable. For instance, there is but little starch in corn until it is perfectly ripe; then the soluble dextrine and sugar are converted into starch and deposited in the kernel for future use. If green corn is eaten we get the starch mostly in soluble form, but as the kernels mature, the dextrin and sugar are finally converted into starch, leaving to remain only a small quantity of sucrose. The same is true of all the cereals.

Nature changes sugar and dextrine in the ripening grain into insoluble starch, and the protoplasmic flour cell contains the food with which the little plant has to start out life in the succeeding generation. But the embryo plant, which again proceeds from the germ, cannot make any use of raw starch; so nature deposits in every kernel of grain, such as wheat, corn, barley, or rye, a little digestive agent, diastase, which has the power of converting the starch into a soluble form, as soon as the sun, moisture and warmth begin their action on the soil. Thus the food is made digestible for the embryo plant, furnishing it with material for building up a stem with its two rudimentary leaves; the plant being nourished in this manner until it grows well above the ground, for only under the vitalizing influence of the direct sunlight is starch formed in the chlorophyll grains by the chemical combination of carbon dioxide and water.

Nature never intended that we should eat products of the soil containing a large amount of raw starch, as our teeth are not suitably constructed for the perfect mastication of dry grain. Persons with sound teeth and healthy digestive organs can undoubtedly eat raw cereals in reasonable amounts with impunity, but it is difficult to break down all the cell walls protecting the starch grains, even by prolonged physical mastication. Only a small percentage of the starch is changed by the enzyme of the saliva; and while the inversion, if there is no hyperacidity, may go on for some time in the stomach, it has to be completed by the more powerful enzyme of the pancreatic juice.

Cereal products should preferably be eaten in a dry state to insure perfect mastication. Mixtures of watery mushes and concentrated cane sugar should be avoided, as they are apt to cause fermentations, because the presence of sugar interferes with the digestion of starch.

Cellulose, an Essential Food Constituent

Cellulose, which also belongs to the class of carbohydrates, is the basis of cell structure of plants and exists in various forms. It is sometimes a hard and dense substance, but in the earlier stages of plant growth, as in tender leaves and vegetables, it is chemically combined with water in a more soluble and digestible form. Until quite recently cellulose was held to be indigestible, but experiments have proved that a large percentage may disappear in the digestive canal, and if the foods are thoroughly masticated from twenty-five to fifty per cent is digested. While, on an average, cellulose may have but little food-value, it is of great importance in acting as a mechanical stimulus to promote the peristaltic movement of the intestine. The diet of man must contain some bulk in the form of more or less woody fibres, as the muscular wall of the intestine, if it has no work to do, becomes atrophied like every other muscle. The lack of cellulose in food is one of the principal causes of constipation.

There is a tendency among the American people to remove as much as possible of the cellulose from food and to give preference to artificially prepared and concentrated food products, a circumstance which has led to an almost universal debility of the intestinal muscular walls, with resultant chronic constipation. For the same reason an exclusive milk diet will lead to costiveness, because animal foods and products contain no cellulose. Whole grain cereals, nuts, vegetables and fruits in their natural state furnish an ample amount of cellulose to promote normal peristaltic movement.

The Pectins

The pectins are jelly-like bodies, which are closely related to those of the carbohydrates and are contained in most fruits and vegetables. In the early stages of growth the pectins are combined with organic acids forming insoluble compounds, but during the ripening of fruit and cooking of vegetables they are changed into soluble compounds, which in nutrition serve practically the same functions as do starches and sugars. In food analyses the pectin bodies are usually included with the carbohydrates.

Fats and Oils, Nature's Lubricants

Fats are nature's most concentrated food principle; they have more than twice the energy value of that released from either proteins or carbohydrates. If taken in moderate quantities in the form of natural foods, fats act as lubricators to the organism as a whole and especially to the intestinal tract.

Fats are found chiefly in the seeds of plants and to some extent in fruits, leaves and stems; also in animal foods, such as milk, eggs and meat. In the animal organism fat is mostly deposited near the surface, but it is also scattered in minute particles through the various tissues. Fats form on an average about fifteen per cent of the weight of the body, but the amount varies with the quantity and quality of foods, exercise, climatic and other conditions. When more food is taken than is necessary for immediate use, the surplus is usually stored up as fat in the body. Lack of certain organic salts, like iron and sodium, in food will also favor the formation of fat, since the blood is unable to take up a sufficient amount of oxygen for the complete combustion of the carbon. Under these conditions, both protein and carbohydrates are converted into adipose tissue.

The fats of the vegetable kingdom are, like the carbohydrates, derived from carbon dioxide and water, and are very likely formed synthetically through the agency of chlorophyll. The fat in the animal body may have three different sources. One portion may be derived from the fats which have been ingested as food. Another portion may be formed from the carbohydrates; while a third portion may result from the decomposition of protein. That portion of the body's fat which is directly derived from the ingested fats is comparatively small, the greater amount resulting from those occurring in the carbohydrates.

The principal fats contained in vegetable and in animal food products are olein, palmitin and stearin. These are chemical combinations of glycerine and fatty acids; the former being a common constituent, while each fat shows its own characteristic acid, such as those known as oleic acid, palmitic acid and stearic acid.

In round numbers it may be said that fats are composed of nine parts of a fatty acid and one part of glycerine. When at a moderate temperature these combinations are in a liquid form they are called oil. If in a solid or semi-solid condition, they are known as fats.

The three fatty acids above mentioned are the most important from a dietetic point of view, as they make up the greater part of the edible vegetable oils and fats. Of the three, oleic acid constitutes the greatest part of nearly all fats, especially of oil. Palmitic acid exists chiefly in certain forms of vegetable oil and fats, while stearic acid is a constituent of animal oils and fats.

The hydrogenation of oils, a process recently discovered, is now widely used for bringing liquid fats into a more or less solid form. The process consists of heating them to a temperature of from 212° F. to 400° F., and of introducing hydrogen in connection with some catalytic agent, such as nickel or platinum. By means of this process the oleic acid molecule takes up two atoms of hydrogen and is turned into stearic acid. After completing the process the metal is removed by filtration. Cotton-seed oil, peanut oil and corn oil are generally hydrogenated, while the oils of olives and nuts are obtained by means of the cold hydraulic pressing of the pulp.

In natural food products the fats are mingled with other substances. Free fats, such as oils (extracted from oily seeds or fruits) and butter, are highly concentrated food principles and should be used sparingly and not without some less concentrated food, such as green-leaf vegetables, which are rich in alkaline bases. In order to be digested, fats must be saponified, i. e., split up in the intestine into glycerine and salts of fatty acids. The presence of free alkalies, especially sodium salts, is necessary for this process of saponification and these are furnished by the bile and pancreatic juice. The fatty acids, after saponification, are absorbed and reconstructed into neutral fats. Fats derived from the vegetable kingdom, including butterfat, should always be preferred to those emanating from various packing houses—lard, margarine, etc. Nuts and such fruits as the olive and avocado are the most hygienic sources of fat, especially nut butters if made from unroasted nuts and brought into a state of emulsion by machinery.

Natural Fruit Acids Do Not Reduce the Alkalinity of the Blood

There prevails an erroneous idea that fruit acids cause acidity of the blood. Acid and sub-acid fruits often cause digestive troubles with people whose blood is in an acid condition from an over-indulgence of meat, cereal foods, sugar, salt, spices, etc., and consequently suffer from a chronic inflammation of the stomach and intestines.

Fruit acids are used by plants in their synthetic processes. In the ripening of fruits some of the acids are utilized in the formation of ethers and carbohydrates, while others are combined to form salts of potassium, sodium, calcium, magnesium, etc. In the latter case these salts are generally changed in the human body into alkaline carbonates, thereby increasing the alkalinity of the blood, digestive juices and glandular secretions. The uncombined acids either form alkaline carbonates, or are oxidized into carbon dioxide and water. Under normal conditions fruit acids increase the alkalinity of the blood, rather than diminish it. Those who suffer from an acid condition and inflammation of the digestive organ can improve their condition by eating plenty of green-leaf vegetables, either slightly steamed or in the form of combination salads. At the same time the amount of meat, eggs and cereals have to be reduced to a minimum, while refined sugar, salt, condiments, coffee and tea must be avoided altogether.

The fruit acids like the sugars and starches, are composed of three elements —carbon, hydrogen and oxygen. They must be distinguished from the products of decomposition and oxidation like uric acid, butyric acid, sulphuric acid, phosphoric acid, which are the result of a high protein diet. These acids must be neutralized and eliminated by the alkaline mineral elements in vegetables and fruits. The principal fruit acids are:

Citric acid, which exists in the free state in many fruits. If combined with alkaline salts, it forms citrates, which are constituents of all the citrus foods, quinces, currants, gooseberries, strawberries, raspberries, cranberries and many others.

Malic Acid occurs in a free state in apples, pears, quinces, sour cherries, pineapple, grapes, currants, blackberries, etc., or in combination with alkaline bases, as malates, in sweet-cherries, apples, rhubarb, gooseberries, grapes and strawberries. Malic acid and citric acid are formed together in unripe apples, grapes, pineapples, gooseberries, cherries, strawberries, etc. Malic acid, or malates, are also found in small quantities in potatoes, carrots and parsley.

Tartaric acid is one of the most common organic acids, especially occurring in grapes and in other fruits.

Gallic acid is widely distributed in vegetables, especially in the form of compounds called tannins.

Oxalic acid occurs throughout the vegetable kingdom, sometimes in the form of oxalate. Sorrel, spinach, rhubarb, cocoa, black tea and pepper contain from two to four per cent in the fresh state. Contrary to the popular opinion, tomatoes show a very small amount, less than 0.005 per mille.

Oxalic acid, when taken in food, circulates through the animal tissues and fluids either as the free acid or as a salt, usually calcium salt. In the normal and healthy body it undergoes oxidation into carbon dioxide and water. In case of high acidity of the blood, a part of the oxalic acid may pass into the kidneys unchanged, giving rise to the formation of calcium oxalates—stones in the kidneys and bladder. The amount of oxalic acid in cocoa and black tea is especially high.

Lactic acid, which is formed during the fermentation of milk sugar or lactose, as in souring of milk, cheese making, and in ripening of cream. Lactic acid is also found as a by-product in the fermentation of various sugars and other substances in the presence of protein.

Formic acid is present in minute quantities in honey. This acid is not contained in the original nectar, but is a product of the glandular secretions of the bee. Formic acid is supposed to act as a preservative and to prevent fermentation.

Tannic acid is found in the skins of fruits and in very small proportions in honey. It also has a preservative action.

CHAPTER IX

THE MINERAL ELEMENTS

The Building Stones of the Body — "The Missing Link in Dietetics"

Although the mineral elements make up only a comparatively small amount of the body—about five per cent—they are nevertheless essential constituents, and every single element has some distinct physiological function to perform. The normal and healthy development of the organism primarily depends upon the adequate supply of the mineral salts, which truly may be called "the building stones of the body."

A normal man weighing 150 pounds is composed of the following 34 or more elements:

90 lbs. oxygen	3½ oz. of sulphur
36 lbs. carbon	3 oz. of potassium
14 lbs. hydrogen	2½ oz. of sodium
3 lbs. 8 oz. of nitrogen	2 oz. of fluorine
3 lbs. 12 oz. calcium	1½ oz. of magnesium
1 lb. 14 oz. of phosphorus	¼ oz. of silicon
4 oz. of chlorine	1/6 oz. of iron

Traces of the following elements: Manganese, aluminum, iodine, arsenic, nickel, copper, lead, zinc, lithium, cobalt, bromine, lanthanum, neodymium, cerium, vanadium, chromium, boron, rubidium, strontium, molybdenum, argon, beryllium, helium, neon, scandium and titanium.

The principal acid-binding or alkaline elements are: Potassium, Sodium, Calcium, Magnesium, Iron, Manganese, Copper, Aluminum.

The principal acid-forming elements are: Phosphorus, Sulphur, Silicon, Chlorine, Fluorine, Iodine, Arsenic.

The Ocean, The Source of Many Elements

As life originated in the sea, which contains nearly all the known elements, we may assume that other elements besides those mentioned are connected with the various life processes. They are probably identified with the origin of chlorophyll and protoplasm itself as the presence of the various chemical elements, in even infinitesimal quantities, is absolutely essential for the growth and physiological functions of the cells; minor deficiencies or entire absence may become detrimental to their development. These problems are certainly opening up great fields of investigation for the biological chemist.

The principal minerals found in sea-water are:

	AVERAGE PER 1000 PARTS
Common salt (sodium chloride)	27.20
Magnesium chloride	3.80
Magnesium sulphate	1.65
Gypsum (calcium sulphate)	1.25
Potassium sulphate	0.86
Calcium carbonate	0.12
Magnesium bromide	0.07

Modern analysis reveals the existence of at least 40 of the 90 known elements in sea-water. It is a well known fact that blood serum and sea-water resemble each other in chemical composition. Our body cells are surrounded by almost the same fluid, as occur in the first protoplasmic formations which floated in the primeval sea.

The arc spectra of the ash of blood always show silver, aluminum, calcium, copper, iron, potassium, sodium, magnesium, manganese, phosphorous, silicon, titanium and zinc. Other elements sometimes found are cobalt, chromium, cerium, lead, nickel, tin and strontium. When the albumins are coagulated by heat, silver, calcium, copper, manganese, nickel, lead, tin and zinc are concentrated, while aluminum and titanium are diminished.

Elements Found in Human Organs

Studies on the ash of organs indicate a concentration of *nickel, cobalt* and *lead* in the pancreas, of *tin* in the suprenal capsules and of *zinc* in the liver and kidneys.

Silver is found principally in the uterus, ovaries and thyroid, with a trace in the heart, spleen and kidneys. *Aluminum* accumulates in the lungs, kidneys and heart, with traces in the testicles and pancreas. *Cobalt* and *nickel* are also present in the pancreas with traces in the other organs. *Chromium* is found in traces in all organs, with a bit more in the thyroid and spleen. *Copper* is abundant in the lungs, liver and heart, with traces in the other organs. *Tin* is abundant in all organs, particularly in the brain, spleen and thyroid. *Titanium* is found in the lungs and only in small traces in other organs. *Zinc* is the principal constituent in the genital organs and thyroid, with traces in other organs, except the heart.

In a group of marine products including fish, crustacea, and sea plants, the following elements were detected by spectroscope in considerable amounts: calcium, iron, magnesium, potassium and sodium. Traces of aluminum, chromium, copper, lead, lithium, manganese and strontium were found in all of the products, while traces of fluorine, nickel, silicon, silver, tin, titanium and zinc were present in some of the products. Columbium and vanadium were doubtfully present, while traces of barium were found in nearly all the products. Boron was detected only in kelp meal.

The Catalytic Action of Elements

A number of the elements enter the body in exceedingly small quantities, because of their presence in food material as one part in a million, or even less. They are none the less essential in speeding up chemical reactions, which otherwise would proceed slowly. About a hundred years ago the Swedish chemist Berzelius, while studying the process of fermentation of sugar in liquids, traced it to the action of a ferment which accelerates the chemical action. He says in part in his report of his investigations:

"Comparing it with known relations in the inorganic world it was seen to be mostly like the quick decomposition of hydrogen peroxide under the influence of platinum, silver, or fibrin; it was, therefore, natural to suppose that the action of the ferment was an analogous one.

"I will call it the *catalytic* power of substances, and the decomposition thereby, *catalysis,* just as we understand by analysis the separation of the constituents of substances by means of affinity. Catalytic power appears to consist essentially in the fact that substances are able to set into activity affinities which are dormant at this particular temperature, and this, not by their own affinity, but by their presence alone.

"We have justifiable reasons to suppose that, in living plants and animals, thousands of catalytic processes take place between the tissues and the liquids in the formation of a great number of dissimilar compounds, for whose formation out of the common raw materials, plant juice or blood, no probable cause could be assigned. The cause will perhaps in the future be discovered in the catalytic power of the organic tissues of which the organs of the living body consist."

Thus Berzelius foresaw the wonderful catalytic power of the elements in building up the organic world, their necessity in the processes of digestion, assimilation and elimination in the animal and human body, their importance in the proper functions of the glands, in fact in all the physiological functions.

Sea Plants a Source of Catalysts

The normal growth of the human organism, its freedom from disease, seems to depend largely on the presence of many elements which have been treated so far as unimportant or have been regarded as accidental in our food and tissues. The importance of a large number of elements in the soil for the healthy growth of plants and trees is likewise apparent. As large areas of land have been depleted of many essential minerals by leaching the soil or by wrong methods of fertilization, attention has been paid within recent years to the utilization of the vegetation of the sea, as accessory foods to the human and animal dietary. If properly prepared, seaplants can be made digestible, thus supplying many minerals which are lacking in the foods grown on impoverished soil.

When the land first appeared in the early geological periods of our planet, it was rich in minerals and could support a giant flora and animal world. But gradually as the epochs passed and every rainfall washed more and more of the elements out of the land and back into the sea, the giant forms of the organic world either disappeared or were reduced in size.

The Dietetic Value of Sea Plants

I am quoting the following from the Scientific American, issue for August, 1931:

"Modern scientists became interested some time ago in the fact that there was a noticeable absence of the deficiency diseases everywhere in the world where sea plants are used for food—Japan, China, Ireland, and all along the northern seas. Interesting himself in a study of this subject, one of the prominent experts on live-stock feeding went to Europe. He was looking for an answer to the problems facing stockmen in certain sections of the United States —diseases, still-births, difficulty in raising the young—and he wanted to study conditions over there.

"He learned among other things that the peasants of some of the countries bordering the seas were in the habit of gathering the sea mosses, drying them in the sun, and then adding them to the cattle's feed. Wherever that was done he observed strong, healthy live-stock. It was a practice worth following up.

"Still with no thought of human dietary needs he returned from Europe and began a search for seaweed that could be fed to animals. The Atlantic coast offered some *dulse* in limited quantities, but on the Pacific coast he found some beds of kelp which had been used during the World War by the Government as a source of potash, iodine and acetone. They were *Macrocystis pyrifera* 'groves' and they extend 200 miles along the coast of Southern California.

"Having introduced kelp to the live-stock with satisfactory results, its promoters began to think of using it for humans, and so a series of white rats from the laboratories of the California State University was called upon to test its efficacy.

"After two years' careful work with the rats, men and women in widely separated areas were selected to test the seaweed, now ground into a fine powder and not unpleasant to the taste. They were individuals suffering from all kinds of diseases. They took the kelp regularly for several months and while there were instances where no apparent results were experienced, benefit in most cases was notable. Every one of the patients who had been suffering from deficiency diseases was benefited to a remarkable degree.

"Analyses of kelp were made by Government chemists from the Department of Agriculture, as well as by chemists in several of the leading universities. The presence of 32 of the chemical elements has already been demonstrated in it and Professor George W. Cavanaugh, head of the Department of Agricultural Chemistry of Cornell, who has spent the past six months studying the plant and its value as a food, states that he is of the opinion that he may find many more of the known elements in it."

Analyses of Foods
Mineral Salts, the Real Materia Medica

The tables of analyses in the appendix show the proportion of mineral elements entering into the composition of the human body and most of the generally used food materials. We see at a glance that there is a variation in the quantity and proportion of the different elements. The green-leaf vegetables have the highest amount of alkaline elements, especially sodium, calcium and iron, which are essential for the formation of normal and healthy blood. On the other hand, the milling products like white flour, bolted corn meal, polished rice, etc., are poorest in the total amount of mineral elements, especially in the amount of the essential blood salts.

The organic salts enter the system as fully oxidized compounds and, therefore, furnish practically no heat energy. Nevertheless, they hold the key to nearly all of the material manifestations of life. They are the builders of sound and normal cells and tissues, giving them firmness and form. They are catalyctic promoters of chemical reactions. It is characteristic of catalysts that they exert their power in very small amounts. One part of catalyst in a million or ten million may be sufficient to hasten significantly the cause of chemical reactions.

They are the essential factors to digestion and assimilation, as ingredients of the digestive juices regulating the osmotic exchange between lymph and blood and cells. They are indispensable in the formation of the secretions of the ductless glands, or hormones, which probably regulate nearly all of the vital processes of the body.

They are the scavengers of the body and purifiers of the blood, neutralizing the waste products, uric acid, carbonic acid, etc., and assisting in removing them from the system. They are the real *materia medica,* which remove one of the fundamental causes of diseases, *toxemia,* and which restore the equilibrium of perfect health; they are nature's real antitoxins, giving vital resistance to every cell and thus making the system invulnerable to all so-called "germs of disease." The knowledge of the actions and reactions of the mineral elements of the body is the foundation upon which a natural system of living and healing must be built.

This branch of food chemistry has received only recently the degree of attention which it deserves, and it may be aptly called *"the missing link in dietetics."* It is a most significant fact that medical textbooks pay very little attention to the importance of mineral elements in the body. No system of cure can be complete and efficient which does not give paramount consideration to the mineral elements in food. The laws of life and growth are closely interwoven with the characteristics of the elements. *The problems of healthy and adequate nutrition cannot be satisfactorily solved without the most extensive and careful study of the physiological functions of all the mineral salts, and their relation in the system to each other.*

The phosphate of lime and the carbonate of lime of the skeleton, the iron contained in the red blood corpuscles, the phosphate of sodium, chloride of potassium, chloride of sodium, etc., found in the blood serum, are organized, and as such they have a certain duration of life during which they have vital functions to perform. Sooner or later the molecules will become fatigued or devitalized, according to the degree of their physiological activity, and they must be supplanted by fresh material. In other words, their biological existence is at an end when the vitality of the molecules imparted to them by the organism of the plant is used up, just as the death of the whole organism occurs when its vitality is exhausted.

To illustrate: the comparatively stable molecules in the bones and teeth will last a longer time before they require replacement than will the highly active atoms of iron, which are the oxygen carriers of the blood. The quantity of blood of a normal adult man of 160 pounds is about twelve pounds (7½ per cent of the body weight) and contains approximately fifty grains of iron. With every pulse beat nearly six ounces of blood are forced from the heart into the lungs and from there into the arteries and capillaries through the body. Consequently the fifty grains of iron pass through the heart and lungs 120 times an hour and 2880 times a day. Within twenty-four hours, under normal conditions, the fifty grains of iron have to expend the same effort or vital action as 2880x50 grains or more than 20 pounds. For that reason a daily supply of iron is most essential and the economical sources are the green-leaf vegetables and fresh fruits, grown on properly fertilized soil.

Variation of the Percentages of Mineral Elements in the Same Kinds of Foods

In studying tables of food analyses one important fact is generally overlooked, viz.: the wide variations in the chemical composition of the mineral matter in food products of the same kind, as illustrated on a page of the general tables. Thus we see, for instance, in cow's milk a variation of the total mineral matter from 0.35 per cent to 1.21 per cent; in grapes from 0.36 to 0.70 per cent; in potatoes from 0.42 to 1.46 per cent; in peas from 1.76 to 3.49 per cent, while soda, lime and iron vary as follows:

		Soda	*Lime*	*Iron*
In milk	from	8.60 to 11.18	17.31 to 27.55	0.33 to 0.76
In grapes	from	0.29 to 10.54	1.70 to 22.60	0.05 to 1.68
In potatoes	from	none to 16.93	0.51 to 6.23	0.04 to 7.18
In peas	from	none to 3.54	2.31 to 7.90	none to 3.83

Again, according to Watts and other chemists, oxide of iron shows the following variations in different cereals:

Percentages of iron in total amount of mineral matter:

In wheat	from trace to 3.3
In oats	from 0.1 to 5.1
In rye	from none to 2.2
In barley	from 0.1 to 2.1
In millet	from trace to 1.8
In rice	from none to 1.4
In corn	from 0.5 to 0.8

Similar variations could very likely be detected in all food products grown in different soils or produced by different methods of fertilization. Such changes may go on slowly and imperceptibly; but in the course of years the soil may deteriorate to such a degree that its products may become of an inferior quality, especially deficient in the essential organic salts. Men and animals subsisting on such abnormal foods will eventually show various signs of degeneration which reveal themselves in defective development of bones and tissues and in the lack of vital resistance.

Polaric Distribution of the Elements

The early agricultural chemists had already found that in plants as well as in animals and man, the mineral elements are not equally distributed, but that certain elements predominate in certain parts of the organism. Thus potassium, sodium, iron and sulphur generally pass into the stems, leaves and fruits of the plants, while potassium, phosphorus and magnesium are the principal mineral constituents of the seeds and roots. This fact becomes apparent by a careful study of the tables of analyses contained in this book. The tendency of certain elements to accumulate in certain parts of the plants may be compared with the polaric distribution of the earth's magnetism which is strongest at its poles. This is probably due to the polaric accumulation of iron which is the principal source of magnetic power on our planet. Just as magnetic iron attracts the non-magnetic metal, so the mineral elements in the living organism of the plant, charged as they are with vital electricity and magnetism by the great central station of the sun, attract similar non-magnetic elements as well as carbon dioxide and ammonia. The latter, combined with water, form the carbohydrates, proteids and nucleo-proteids. We may always recognize in plants distinct parts or poles, characterized by the particular mineral elements which they attract and accumulate, viz.: the leaves, blades, stems and juicy fruits on one hand, and on the other, the seeds (grains, nuts, seeds contained in fruits) which served for the reproduction of the species. The polaric distribution can also be noticed to a certain extent in the seeds themselves. Here we find in the outer layer of the kernels an accumulation of calcium, sodium, magnesium, sulphur, fluorine and silica, while potassium and phosphorus predominate in the inner parts. Even in the cells a characteristic division of the elements in the cell walls from the interior parts can be detected.

In the human and animal bodies nature works according to the same principle. Here we find the same anatomical parts—the muscular tissues, the cartilage, the skeleton, the blood, the organs, etc.—likewise characterized by the polaric accumulation of certain mineral elements. The muscular tissues of meat, being rich in potassium and phosphorus, resemble in their chemical composition those of the seeds, while the skeleton, blood and skin, with their large amount of calcium, sodium, magnesium, iron, silicon, chlorine and fluorine, may be compared with the stems, leaves and juicy fruits. Although sodium, chlorine and iron predominate in the blood, the latter must necessarily carry a certain quantity of all the elements entering into the composition of the human body, because it is blood which carries them to the different parts and organs, nourishing and cleansing the tissues and creating heat, vital electricity and magnetism.

ORGANIC VERSUS INORGANIC SALTS

As Revised by
LILLIAN R. CARQUE
NATURAL BRANDS RESEARCH FOUNDATION

Important biochemical findings disclose that the fixed line of demarcation between organic and inorganic minerals is not sharply defined or established as so many dietitians, naturopaths and others erroneously suppose. It is true that the higher the forms of life and the more intense the vital activity of the elements in the organism, the more subtle and refined their organic combinations have to be.

The long-standing and popular belief, still prevailing, is that the chemical elements in inorganic form evolve into organic combinations after they become an intrinsic part of plant structure, and only in this latter state of evolution are they or can they be assimilated by the blood or utilized in the body. According to the late Dr. William Schuessler's Biochemic System of Medicine, there is no difference, per se, in the mineral particle itself from the moment it is picked up from the soil by the capillary attraction or suction, created by the action of cosmic electricity or life, until it passes into the structure of the plant, and finally is drawn into the blood stream where it is carried off by the blood absorbents. Dr. Victor K. LaMer, Associate Professor of Chemistry at Columbia University, New York City, stated in the Literary Digest's issue for August 13, 1932, that "contrary to the preconceived opinion, the inorganic salts *are utilized by the blood the same as are those in food.*" (*Italics ours*)

The following is a perfect analogy: The bricks in a pile on the sidewalk are INorganic before being used or put together, whereas the bricks in a building are organic, because they have been united or *organized*. As individual units, people come together to take part in a certain movement which is termed an organization, but per se they are not changed. Thus it can be seen that there is no difference between organic and inorganic minerals than that which exists between a piece of lumber or a brick lying on the sidewalk or after the material has been fastened into place with nails or held together with cement. In like manner, the plant consists of tiny, practically microscopic mineral particles drawn into their proper positions in the cells to form the building or plant structure. It is exactly as if an invisible mason carried them there and placed them into position with his own hands. Before being so placed, they may be termed INorganic, and after having been assembled, they become organic, because organized.

Many nutritionists admit that chemically and physically elements are always the same, whether they are found in the air, earth, plant or animal. They are none the less inflexible in their opinion that a vital change occurs in all chemical elements as they pass from the mineral kingdom into the structure of the plant, and finally when they become integral parts of the living body; and that their rates of vibration differ according to their scale of evolution. Some dietitians even yield the point that the elements in their inorganic form may be absorbed by the human lacteals and may enter into circulation; they may even produce some chemical changes or reactions, but they repudiate their efficacy in performing any vital functions, due to their lack of the imponderable vital electricity and magnetism which is imparted to them in the organic combinations of the vegetable kingdom.

The vibratory law of all material manifestations and of all relationships does not imply that mineral elements, per se, undergo a process of transmutation, i. e., that they are brought into a higher rate of vibration as they pass from the inorganic to the organic state. The atomic vibration of a chemical element is of necessity always the same; it never changes. It always creates in the ether a wave of the same definite length and by this it is identified. Each substance has its own rate of motion. Thus phosphate of potassium has the highest rate of vibration or motion of any of the mineral substances in the body. It is equally correct to say that we name a specific rate of motion or energy potassium phosphate.

The only difference is in the *size of the particles of minerals,* not in the minerals themselves. The cells of the body utilize those of a certain size or mesh; when they are too large, the blood corpuscles cannot absorb them. The finer or smaller-sized are the particles of minerals, the more do they attract from the atmosphere increased etheric essence. The great mass of inorganic minerals that enter the human or animal organism act as irritants because their massiveness prohibits them from being appropriated, their particles often being larger than is the cell.

Thorough mastication and the digestive processes are not able to break up inorganic minerals into their original atoms. Thus pulverizing is necessary before the cell can attract and assimilate them. That is why a crude inorganic mineral is useless unless the atoms are liberated; they must have room to act, namely to vibrate. If mineral elements are coarse when they enter the body, as compared with other particles that are finer, they retain that degree of density and pass out of the organism unabsorbed, or remain as an irritant or as a foreign body

Nor do high degrees of heat as employed in cooking, baking and frying kill or reduce organic minerals to their more stable inorganic state. The life and consistency of the minerals are not affected at all; they often do pass into the water in which foods are cooked and are lost if the vegetables are drained—that is all. Cooked foods, of course, do undergo a coagulation of certain substances in the protoplasm, albumin or proteid content; the latter contain various coagulable matters which solidify or thicken at different temperatures, ranging from 140 to 200 Fahrenheit. A temperature sufficient to decompose protein matter, if sufficiently prolonged, demolishes the highly intricate molecular structure upon which vegetable life depends, thus disorganizing or separating many organic mineral compounds from their subtle protoplasmic structures.

The breaking up of inorganic minerals into an impalpable powder, so fine as to be scarcely sensed on the tongue, is accomplished best by subjecting inorganic minerals to a continuous process of trituration until the molecules of the salts become diffused evenly throughout the triturating medium and attain homeopathic attenuation. Thus, without the aid of physical phenomena, the biochemist achieves, by the mechanics of grinding his crude minerals, a triturated consistency equally as high as that which is effected naturally by the elaboration of sunlight, water, air and the elements of the soil in the physiology of plant growth. Homeopathic laboratories then proceed to mix thoroughly certain minerals with sugar of milk and to press them into tablets, thus rendering them available for internal use to supply deficiencies in the human organism.

For best results, no one specific inorganic mineral is used alone. Biochemists therefore combine the proper quantity of a kindred chemical into the union of sodium chloride, iron phosphate, sodium phosphate, lime phosphate or chloride of potassium, etc. Taken in an uncombined or elementary state, most elements would be more or less injurious or even poisonous to the system, on account of their great affinity for oxygen and other elements, which rapidly disintegrate all organized matter. It is only in their various chemical combinations with other substances that the elements become so modified that they can serve as sustenance for plants, animals and humans.

The great mass of evidence based on the feeding of animal and human subjects both supports and opposes the absorption of inorganic minerals. This leads us to believe that the crude chemicals that gave unsatisfactory results when ingested were not properly compounded with kindred minerals in correct proportions, or were not broken up into the needed trillions of particles essential to be small enough to serve as living storage batteries. In no instance did these feeding experiments disclose the consistency of the inorganic minerals nor the degree of trituration, and not unlikely inorganic iron or sulphur, for example, was administered alone uncompounded with other minerals of natural affinity.

In all likelihood the experimental feeding tests which reflect discredit on the biochemical need for inorganic minerals may be due, in part, to a preponderance of foods used which were high in the specific organic minerals under observation, and which were probably grown on properly fertilized soil. Since the body absorbs only that which serves its immediate physiological needs in most instances, it obviously eliminates many superfluous elements through the normal channels of excretion. Thus no improvement was registered in many tests by the added ingestion of inorganic minerals.

The following excerpts taken from highly accredited authoritative sources are unbiased, and substantiate the evidence herein set forth, in an endeavor to redeem the reputation of the grossly maligned inorganic minerals:

Professor Henry C. Sherman in his CHEMISTRY OF FOOD AND NUTRITION quotes an experimenter Marshall (Journal of the American Medical Association, Vol. 64, page 573; 1915) thus: "Marshall considers the evidence fully sufficient to warrant the conclusion that organic phosphorus compounds are of no more value as food than are the inorganic phosphates."

In the NEWER KNOWLEDGE OF NUTRITION by McCollum and Simmonds (3rd edition) it states on page 359: "In recent years numerous successful experiments involving growth by Osborne and Mendel (1918) and by McCollum and Simmonds, and others, have repeatedly demonstrated that inorganic compounds of sodium, potassium, calcium, magnesium, chlorin, iodine, phosphorus and iron may be assimilated by animals when no other sources of these elements are provided."

John Aulde, M. D., in his CALCIUM THERAPY (page 78) states: "Organic salts take no precedence over the inorganic, since it has been shown that absorption and therapeutic effect are equally as prompt and efficient whatever salt is selected for administration, and the efficiency depends upon thorough trituration."

Based on feeding tests with clients over a period of twenty years, the Carey-Perry School of the Chemistry of Life in Hollywood, California, reports that "when natural foods are supplemented by inorganic mineral salt tablets, the latter enter the blood *before* those in the food, because the former must first be freed by the digestive processes. For when the liver, stomach and other glands pertaining to digestion refuse to function, as is the case in acute dyspepsia; or when the kidneys cease to work due to uremic poisoning, thus preventing the blood from receiving organized salts or minerals, relief is obtained when the blood is supplied by the supplemented inorganic salts." It is here where inorganic mineral compounds, properly triturated, exert their most salutary influence. Under such adverse conditions, the blood otherwise would become rapidly impoverished, in addition to its already deficient condition.

Sodium Chloride

(Common Table Salt)

As Revised by

LILLIAN R. CARQUE

Nutritionists, lecturers and doctors in the health movement have repeatedly emphasized that the craving for common table salt (sodium chloride) is a result of a perverted taste, that salt serves no purpose as food, nor does it perform any vital functions in the organism. Many authorities are firm in their conviction that a natural diet predominating in green leafy vegetables, if rationally prepared, furnish all the necessary sodium and chlorine for proper nutrition. Especially is this so where foods are grown on properly fertilized soil, and where Pacific Ocean Kelp (Macrocystis Pyrifera) and Dulse (Sea Lettuce) are contributed to the diet in generous quantities. They maintain—and rightfully so—that salt is used in an attempt to restore the organic salts dissolved in the water, foolishly discarded, in which vegetables were boiled, or lost by other irrational methods of preparing foods.

It is also emphasized that common table salt leaves the body in a totally unaltered condition, proving that it remains unabsorbed in the organism, and hence there is no physiological necessity for it. It is likewise deplored that salt does create an unnatural thirst, as it deprives the tissues of a large amount of water on account of its diuretic properties. Thus it stimulates the kidneys to excessive excretions of urine which constantly carry off essential mineral elements from blood and lymph, imposing at the same time unnecessary work on the emunctories.

Let us now examine the facts in the other side of the case, as elucidated in a most unique treatise under title of THE ZODIAC AND THE SALTS OF SALVATION by Dr. Carey and Inez Eudora Perry:

> "With the exception of phosphate of lime, the human system contains more sodium chloride than any other inorganic salt. The reason for this may be readily understood when we realize that our bodies are about 90 per cent water, which in the absence of sodium chloride would be inert and useless. It is the power that this salt has to use water that renders it of any value to man. The same holds good in plants and vegetable life.
>
> "The blood serum is the saline (sea water) solution which vitalizes the blood corpuscles swimming in it. This serum is, therefore, the salt sea of the body in which live the physiological FISH, for the CORPUSCLES ARE FISH IN THE HUMAN SEA.
>
> "As fish, which are natural habitants of salt water, cease living when removed from it, so do the physiological fish die when sodium chloride falls far below its normal quantity.
>
> "It is a fact that this salt does absorb water, but it is not its first or basic nature. Indeed, it possesses a far more subtle and portentous attribute. It has the power to ATTRACT water, therefore *actually to draw it to itself—to become one with it.*
>
> "There are many who either do not care for water, or are unable to retain it long after drinking it. This is easily explained by the fact that the cells of the body do not contain sufficient sodium chloride particles to *attract* water. Hence, when it enters the stomach, they are not present to seize upon and carry it around and distribute to the parts requiring it.
>
> "Lack of thirst—no desire to drink water—arises from the same cause. When a sufficient number of Natrium mur (sodium chloride) particles are present, their call for water manifests in thirst, and constitutes a decided chemical pull. The human body slowly becomes parched and dry when this much-needed salt diminishes in quantity."

Obviously common table salt is largely unassimilable because it consists, for the most part, of crude particles too coarse or large to be taken up by the red blood corpuscles. That is why the blood is unable to obtain the quantity needed—a condition aggravated by serious soil deficiencies, which menace our natural foods and present a nutritional stumbling block to conscientious health seekers. But there are many tiny ones that are absorbed, which are craved and consumed with avidity. This probably explains the tendency to overindulge in salty foods or in common salt as seasoning, far in excess of physiological needs.

It is in all likelihood, too, the impoverished condition of the soil that sets up a painful craving for salt in herbivorous animals who search for salt licks, which craving is sensed equally as keenly by many vegetarians. Carnivora and Eskimos display a repugnance to salted foods because they utilize the blood, the organs, along with the bones and flesh of their prey. Much salt is lost from the body in free perspiring. Consequently, there has to be a supply to make up this abnormal loss. Obviously, for this reason Eskimos do not crave salt.

It is idle to deny that the unassimilated coarse particles often act as an irritant in the stomach and intestinal tract, but where inorganic sodium chloride is not crude, but triturated to homeopathic potency as elsewhere explained, the blood corpuscles can and do absorb them. Fortunately tablets of this specially processed sodium chloride combined with sugar of milk are now available.

We also communicated with large west-coast evaporators of Pacific Ocean Salt in an endeavor to persuade them to see the wisdom of reducing sodium chloride into an impalpable powder that pours, and of making it available at low cost. Their representative assured us that while it was obligatory that other inorganic minerals be triturated to homeopathic attenuation to permit their solubility with bodily fluids, such was not the case with common table salt (sodium chloride) because of its natural affinity for water. He then proceeded to immerse in separate glasses of water both coarse-grained and finely-particled lumps of salt and both were equally soluble, the coarse salt perhaps taking a little longer to become saturated with the fluid. His obvious conclusion was that transgressors are never moderate salt eaters; that doctors who emphasize the deleterious consequences of salt eating see the worst cases—the human wrecks; that the 90 per cent fluidic content of the organism was equal to the task of dissolving a moderate amount of salt ingested; and that danger lurked in a daily intake of salt to a point of saturation or beyond the bodily fluids' capacity to insure complete solubility.

To this Biochemist Inez Eudora Perry, co-author quoted elsewhere in this treatise, comments: "You did not see the salts dissolve in *bodily fluids, but in water*. Don't you see that bodily fluids are different because of their deficiencies? Besides the character of fluids varies. As you know, if you will study a chemical dictionary, *different kinds of fluids create solubility*. Complete solubility is possible only in a normal body, and as we don't know anyone who is normal it is difficult to judge. Some people scarcely have anywhere near enough fluids to dissolve the coarse salt. When deficiencies of potassium chloride and silicon occur, the blood tends to thicken; and hence salt particles are not dissolved rapidly enough.

"Under such adverse conditions, the bodies vary in their fluidic content and it is thus impossible for a full quota of salt to be supplied to the blood stream. Water is picked up and carried to the cells and elsewhere only through the agency of sodium chloride, the water-bearer. It is therefore self-evident that ALL ingested common table salt is not made available for the cells, because this CARRIER of water would insure sufficient bodily fluids if the needed sodium chloride was present in assimilable form. Biochemically triturated sodium chloride is so prepared that it is readily absorbed by the blood corpuscles, despite any undesirable thickness created by congestions or swellings.

"Moreover, the fact that people consume enormous quantities of salt and STILL CRAVE MORE is indubitable proof that, for some reason or other, the salt consumed is not entering the blood, and I claim that the particles are far too large. When the biochemically triturated sodium chloride is taken over a period of time, one will not crave it as formerly. This is more noticeable in winter when one does not perspire so much and thus loses less salt that way."

Let us hope that the salt industries will earnestly consider the imperative need for triturated sodium chloride to insure and hasten complete absorption, and thus render more accessible to the blood serum an adequate supply of severely needed saline fluids. There is also less danger of coarse salt lodging in the organism unassimilated, and serving only as an irritant. Meanwhile a reduction in the consumption of coarse inorganic table salt is advocated, and an increased intake of those foods and nutritional adjuncts predominating in sodium and chlorine, fortified by salt substitutes abounding in such corrective mineral constituents.

CHAPTER X

THE ACID-BINDING OR ALKALINE ELEMENTS

The principal acid-binding, or alkaline elements, necessary for the growth of the human body, and the performance of its physiological functions, are potassium, sodium, calcium, magnesium, iron, copper, manganese, zinc, nickel and aluminum.

Potassium

Potassium exists in inorganic nature in the form of chloride and sulphate of potassium in sea-water, or as deposits of rock salt in the earth's crust; it is also found as silicate of potassium in feldspar and glimmer. Seeds always contain much more potassium phosphate than sodium phosphate, while the proportion of soda to potash is found to be largely in the leaves and in a number of roots.

Phosphate of potassium is the mineral basis of all muscular tissues, giving them their characteristic pliancy. All other organic salts exist in muscular tissues only in small proportions. Meat is a very incomplete food, aside from the objection of waste products it contains. It is adapted only to carnivorous animals, which are able to get their supply of soda, lime and iron by devouring the blood, bones and cartilage of their prey. Cereals, especially white flour products, show the same deficiency in organic salts as does meat. Although the saying, "There is no life where there is no potassium," cannot be contradicted, it must be modified to the extent that potassium acts more favorably when the other elements are present in right proportions.

Potassium is essential not only in the formation of carbohydrates and fat, but also in that of proteids, which are the principal organic compounds of the plant cell. In the synthetic processes of animal life, potassium salts are also indispensable. They play a part in the formation of glycogen from glucose, of fats from glycogen, and of proteids from peptones and proteoses. The liver, which is the principal organ in glycogen-formation, contains twice as much potassium as sodium, while in the spleen the proportion of potassium to sodium is one to four. Potassium is also a predominant element in the red blood corpuscles and in the brain, and we may conclude, therefore, that the element is in some way concerned in the generation of vital electricity and in the functions of the brain and nervous system. Although potassium and sodium have similar chemical properties, they cannot be replaced by each other.

Sodium

A Solvent and Eliminator

Sodium occurs in organic nature in the form of salts, generally as chloride of sodium in the water of oceans and salt seas, and to a smaller extent, in spring waters. It exists as common salt in the strata of the earth's crust. As nitrate of sodium, or chili-nitre, it is found in large quantities in South America. As silicate of sodium it is a constituent of many minerals.

In the animal and human organism sodium has many important functions to perform. In combination with chlorine it is one of the principal constituents of blood and lymph. For the conduct of the electric induction-current, which is generated in the nerve-spirals by the iron of the blood, a salty liquid is necessary as is shown by the construction of electric batteries. The normal blood serum contains for this purpose a comparatively large quantity of sodium chloride, which favors and sustains the generation and conduction of electric currents.

Sodium further serves to make the lime and magnesia salts in our food and, consequently in the blood, more soluble and to keep them in a liquid state for perfect assimilation. Lime and magnesia, if not kept liquid by sodium, are soon deposited in the body, obstructing the capillaries, causing gall and bladder stones, paralysis, etc. Sodium also protects the blood from becoming too easily coagulated, the same as in the case of milk, where it keeps the casein, which is combined with lime and magnesia, in a liquid state. How very important sodium and sodium salts are for healthy nutrition appears, for instance, in the case of diphtheria. The real cause of this disease is a secretion of fibrin through the fauces from lymph and blood, because the latter does not contain enough sodium salts to prevent rapid coagulation of the fibrin. These salts have the property of re-dissolving even the coagulated fibrin and of reducing it again to its liquid state.

Sodium also plays an important part in the formation of saliva, pancreatic juices and of bile. In the last, especially, the dissolving and reducing properties of the sodium salts can be very distinctly recognized in the emulsification and saponification of fats. Without a sufficient amount of sulphate of soda in our food, no normal bile can be formed, and grave disorders of the digestive functions, such as flatulency and constipation will follow.

The deficiency of sodium in the blood is also one of the principal causes of diabetes, because of the inability of the system to take up sufficient oxygen to burn the carbon in the food.

It has been pointed out that the absorption of oxygen depends on the amount of iron in the hemoglobin of the blood. On the other hand, the excretion of carbonic acid, as a result of the oxidation of protein, fat and carbohydrates, is carried on by the sodium phosphate and sodium carbonate contained in the blood and lymph.

Cereals, pulses and nuts are low in the amount of sodium and should, therefore, form the smaller part of our dietary, while the bulk of our food should consist of fresh fruits and vegetables, giving always preference to those rich in organic sodium salts.

Calcium and Magnesium

The Builders of Bones

Calcium (lime) in nature is always accompanied by more or less magnesium, and, with the former, it represents the opposite pole to potassium (phosphate of potash), which predominate in seeds and in the muscular tissues of the animals, thus holding the balance to these substances. Calcium in connection with magnesium is, therefore, the mineral foundation of the entire skeleton, as well as of the cartilages and tendons. Magnesium gives the bones a certain flexibility and protects them from becoming too easily fractured.

Magnesium occupies a position intermediate between the alkali metals and the alkaline earths. To some extent it also resembles the element zinc. Magnesium is widely diffused in nature and several of its compounds are found in large quantities. It occurs as chloride and sulphate in many spring waters and in the salt mines of Strassfurt (Germany).

Lime and magnesia play also an important part in the vegetable kingdom. Analytical investigations show that lime and magnesia are present in every part of the plant. The leaves contain relatively more lime, and the seeds relatively more magnesia than do other parts of the plants. These characteristics are the result of certain functions. The lime is necessary for the formation of certain calcium compounds of nucleo-proteids required in the organized structures of nuclei and chlorophyll bodies of the leaves, while the magnesium serves for the assimilation of phosphorus acid, as magnesium phosphate can give up its phosphoric acid more easily than any other phosphate that occurs in plant juices. Thus calcium is chiefly required for the construction of plant tissue and at the same time facilitates the assimilation of other elements, while magnesium serves especially in aiding the assimilation of phosphoric acid. These two elements can exert their nutritive functions only while they are in a certain dependence upon each other. An excess of the former in the soil will lead to starvation of the plants, and predominance of the latter to poisonous phenomena in growth. Lime is necessary for the formation of the bones. In fact, a higher development in form and function becomes possible only when the lower forms of life acquire the ability to assimilate lime and to utilize the resulting calcium proteid compound for the formation of nuclei.

Lime, Essential for Plant Growth

A deficiency of lime in the soil makes itself visible in diseased leaves and retarded growth. It has been found that etiolated or pale leaves contain less lime than do greener leaves. According to chemcial analysis, 1,000 parts of green leaves contain 13.3 parts of lime, while the same quantity of etiolated leaves shows only 2.6 parts of lime. Diseased leaves of the sugar beet shows only half the amount of lime present in the healthy leaves. The favorable influence of lime on certain soils has led to the very common agricultural practice of liming.

Magnesium salts are especially important in the formation of seeds which are rich in phosphoric acid, but they are also required by all other parts of plants, especially those in the process of development. Seeds rich in fat contain more magnesia than do those rich in starch. The average proportion of magnesia is polarized in the outer coat or bran, which contains about four times as much of this element as does the whole kernel, and about twenty times as much as occur in the flour cells.

In man and the higher vertebrate animals the lime salts make up more than 50 per cent of all the mineral elements composing the body. They are not only necessary for the formation of bones, but also for every part of the organism. Lime and iron are essential for the production of red blood corpuscles which are essential for proper respiration, since it is their function chemically to combine with oxygen.

Calcium stands for strength and durability in the animal organism. In order to retain health and strength the food should contain the necessary amount of organic lime salts. Without a sufficient amount of lime, firm and healthy bones cannot be built. Even in the adult the bony tissues must be renewed from time to time, as they are subject to change of matter like all the other tissues of the body. Blood vessels enter the bones. They supply them with the necessary material for growth and tissue changes. In this way the bones are furnished with phosphates of lime and the other elements entering into their structure. The arteries and capillaries bring continuously new material for the repair of all parts of the skeleton. On the other hand, the veins constantly carry away some of the worn-out lime salts for excretion. If there is a deficiency of the lime salts in the food, and consequently in the blood, the gelatine of the bones loses its chemical support and begins to decompose. Thus the teeth are first attacked from the inside by the venous blood, becoming hollow, while the saliva attacks them from without, dissolving the gelatinous matter which has lost its hold. In this way the teeth are deprived of their support in both directions and decay prematurely.

Calcium in Relation to Sodium

It is often maintained that foods rich in lime tend to ossify the arteries and cause calcareous degeneration of the tissues. This occurs only in those cases where the blood does not contain sufficient sodium salts to keep the phosphate of lime in solution. That there is a lack of sodium in the usual diet of meat, white flour products and of poorly prepared vegetables, has been pointed out. The increasing consumption of alcoholic beverages, such as wine and beer, likewise the use of vinegar, which are all deficient in mineral elements, also deprive the blood of organic salts, which are carried away by increased urination and by the removal of carbon dioxide resulting from the oxidation of alcohol. When wine and beer are drunk regularly every day, in time a condition must necessarily arrive when the blood does not contain a sufficient amount of the essential organic salts for the formation of red blood corpuscles. It is then that asthma, corpulency and rheumatism appear.

The greater part of the calcium, magnesium and sodium salts are contained in the blood, bones, tendons and cartilages. These are devoured by the carnivorous animals, but are not food for man, who should chiefly derive his supply of these elements from fresh fruits and vegetables. The usual meat and cereal diet, especially white flour products in combination with refined sugar, are wholly inadequate in the amount of the above-named organic salts. A large number of diseases, especially during childhood, where the tissue changes are most pronounced, must be attributed to this fact.

It has been estimated that the calcium requirements of the average adult person are about 0.45 gram or 200 grains per day. This requirement must naturally increase in maternity, especially during the last three months of pregnancy, when the foetus is rapidly growing. A daily supply of green-leaf vegetables in the form of salads is, therefore, absolutely necessary, not only to insure the normal growth of the unborn child, but also an easy parturition.

Magnesium, a Hardener of Bones and Teeth

Magnesium exists in the body principally as phosphate of magnesia in the bones, which contain about 50 per cent of phosphate of lime and one per cent of phosphate of magnesia. Yet this comparatively small quantity gives the skeleton its firmness and prevents softening of the bones, because they contain 1½ per cent or ½ per cent more phopshate of magnesia than do the bones. This explains the fact that in exhumation of ancient skulls the jawbones are partly decayed and decomposed, while the teeth are still pretty well preserved. The ivory tusks of elephants contain two per cent phosphate of magnesium, and the billiard balls made from them are almost indestructible. The teeth of carnivorous animals contain nearly five per cent phosphate of magnesia, and for that reason, they are able to crush and grind the bones of their prey without difficulty.

Magnesium, as well as calcium, iron and sulphur, also take part in the formation of the albumen of the blood. Màgnesium has peculiar vitalizing powers. It predominates over calcium in the muscular tissues, brain and nerves. Normal and healthy lungs show twice as much magnesia as that of lime. We must consider the salts of magnesium as cell-builders, particularly of the nervous system and lung tissues. They are also instrumental in reducing foreign matter and waste, and in carrying them out of the system, assisting the functions of the excretory organs and in maintaining the natural fluidity of the blood and osmotic pressure, without which metabolism would be impossible.

Magnesium salts can exert their nourishing functions only in the presence of calcium salts, while in the absence of the latter they have an injurious effect. The absence of magnesium salts in otherwise complete culture solutions leads to a gradual stoppage of all further development and to final inanition. The determination and balancing of the available amount of magnesia and lime in the soils are therefore, an important factor in successful farming. While lime salts are indispensable for animals, the higher plants and for algae, they are not so in the case of bacteria, fungi and lower algae.

Iron

A Catalyst and Oxidizer

Among all the heavy metals iron is the most useful as well as the most widely and abundantly diffused in nature. It is usually found in small quantities in nearly all forms of rock, clay, sand and earth. It never occurs as a free metal, but chiefly combined with oxygen as ferrous and ferric oxides. In inorganic form iron is generally combined with oxygen, sulphur, carbon and silicon. Silicates of iron, when decomposed by atmospheric carbonic acid, turn into carbonate of iron which is soluble in water containing carbonic acid, and is thus distributed by water all over the earth. Carbonate of iron, in coming in contact with the air, is oxidized into oxide of iron. The latter is again reduced by decaying organic matter into carbonate of iron and is dissolved and carried off by water. We have, therefore, in iron a ceaseless oxidizing agent, preventing the retention of carbon in the soil and enabling it to return to the air, in order to begin anew the cycle of life.

In the organic world iron plays the same important part as a carrier of oxygen and stands in the closest possible relation to the fundamental processes of change of matter or metabolism.

It has been pointed out heretofore that iron in the animal organism does not occur in an inorganic form, but as a small part of a compound. This is the most complicated compound that has been investigated, containing as it does over two thousand atoms in a molecule and making up the red coloring matter of the blood, the hemoglobin, which first appears in the body of the vertebrate animals. The vegetable kingdom, which has the power of assimilating inorganic compounds of iron, builds up the complex organic compounds from which the hemoglobin is produced. Iron is taken from the soil and is carried to the leaves, where it takes part in the formation of the chlorophyll granules, which is the green coloring matter of nature.

If plants are allowed to grow in solutions free from iron, the leaves become colorless or etiolated, but turn green as soon as iron salts are added to the liquid in which the roots are immersed. The amounts of iron and chlorophyll vary in the different parts of the plant. For instance, the green leaves of cabbage contain four times as much iron as do the inner etiolated leaves. From many investigations it appears that in the bodies of plants, animals and man, iron serves for the following distinct purposes:

(1) For the production of the chlorophyll of the plant, principally contained in the green leaves, and of the hemoglobin of the red blood corpuscles.

(2) For the assimilation of carbon dioxide and for the synthesis of

organic matter from inorganic matter in the plant by means of the chlorophyll and sunlight.

(3) For the process of respiration in man and animals. It is the hemoglobin that carries the molecular oxygen through the capillaries to all parts of the body where the ingested food, which has been changed into blood and lymph and stored in the cells of the tissues, is oxidized or burnt.

(4) For the generation of a magnetic blood current and an electromagnetic induction current in the nerve spirals which pass through the walls of arteries and veins and help to build and nourish them.

Chlorophyll, or the coloring matter of the leaf, which also needs for its production other mineral elements besides iron (such as lime and phosphoric acid), is closely related to hemoglobins, or the coloring matter in the blood, and the formation of the latter depends upon the presence of the former. Only those cells in the plant that contain chlorophyll are capable of absorbing carbon dioxide. Without the latter the necessary proteins cannot be formed. as the plant must construct the highly complex protein molecule out of the simplest inorganic compounds, viz: carbon dioxide, water, salts and oxygen, while the animal obtains the organized food without which it cannot live.

The Function of Iron in the Liver and Spleen

The total amount of iron in the human body is comparatively small and probably does not exceed seventy-five grains in the normal state of health. Of this quantity about fifty grains are contained in the blood, the remainder being distributed in the marrow of the bones, the liver and principally in the spleen. Iron is perhaps the most active element in the system and needs, therefore, to be renewed more frequently than do for instance calcium and potassium.

That nature tries to protect the system from a deficiency of iron, by storing this element in the liver and spleen, is a most significant fact. Under normal conditions these organs store up a certain amount of iron to be drawn upon when there is a sudden demand for the rapid formation of red corpuscles, as for instance after heavy losses of blood. In the liver we find iron in various forms, from the simple oxide and phosphate of iron to the more complicated compounds which rapidly diminish after hemorrhages, or when the food does not furnish the requisite amount of this element. This circumstance indicates that the normal liver maintains the balance of organic iron in the system, thus repairing any accidental loss.

Most remarkable and characteristic is the function of iron in the spleen, an organ whose physiological importance has not been understood until recent years. The spleen acts in our system as an electric power station where the blood is recharged with electricity.

While a most comprehensive table of the iron contents of foods is given with the other tables, we shall consider here only some of the most frequently used articles of the human dietary, stating the amount of iron in 1000 parts of water-free substance:

Food	Iron	Food	Iron
Meat of chicken	trace	Pinions	0.60
Fish	trace	Walnuts	0.61
White flour	0.03	Cherries	0.70
Dates	0.03	Carrots	0.70
Polished rice	0.05	Prunes	0.94
Bananas	0.07	Tomatoes	1.00
Human milk	0.07	Horseradish	1.25
Meat, average	0.15	Gooseberries	1.32
Beans	0.19	Rye bran	1.40
Unpolished rice	0.22	Cucumbers	1.40
White of egg	0.25	Pumpkins	1.88
Rye	0.25	Cabbage	2.16
Peanuts	0.27	Onions	2.20
Cow's milk	0.30	Swiss chard	2.30
Whole wheat	0.30	Asparagus	2.94
Wheat bran	0.38	Radishes	3.00
Oranges	0.38	Strawberries	3.73
Cocoanut	0.40	Rice bran	4.00
Yolk of egg	0.40	Spinach	6.05
Grapes, average	0.45	Leeks	7.60
Apples	0.46	Lettuce	9.40
Figs	0.60	Sorrel	9.85

Milk Deficient in Iron

In a series of carefully conducted experiments with animals, the German scientist Bunge has shown that the amount of iron is five times higher in the liver of the new-born than in that of full-grown animals. Nature seems to have made this wise provision for the reason that the organic compounds of iron are apparently assimilated with great difficulty by the new-born. Hence, the material organism uses up its supply of iron with the greatest economy. The amount which may be conveyed to the infant organism could reach it in two ways: through the placenta or through the mammary glands. Nature chooses the former as a safer plan because the organic compounds of iron, if conveyed through the mouth and alimentary canal, might be decomposed by fermentative processes before they could be absorbed by the system. That nature protects the growing organism from a deficiency of iron is certainly proof of the great necessity for an ample supply of this element in building up the normal and healthy body. In the light of this knowledge, it seems very probable that children often become anemic, if the milk diet is prolonged or too exclusively employed after the natural period of lactation.

Diet During Nursing

Only a small quantity of iron is assimilated from the milk during lactation. Bunge showed that in young rabbits the absolute amount of iron remains nearly always the same, while the body increases in weight sixfold by the end of the fourth week. Consequently, the relative proportion of iron falls to one-sixth and the animals at this time appear to be already anemic. As soon as they begin to feed on grass and green leaves containing an abundance of iron, the amount of hemoglobin begins to increase again.

It has been estimated that the normal child at birth has about ten grains of iron, of which two-thirds is drawn from the organism of the mother during the last three months. It is therefore very important that before and during this period the diet should furnish an abundance of iron, as well as sodium and of calcium. During normal lactation the daily secretion of milk is about one quart. The iron requirement of the mother must be increased accordingly by a liberal supply of fresh fruits and vegetables.

Next to milk, cereals, which are so-called staple foods, contain the smallest amount of iron, at least in the form in which they are generally consumed, when deprived of their outer coats. Chemical analysis shows that white flour and polished rice contain only one-half as much iron as does human milk, and rice even ten times less than does cow's milk. All grains contain iron, which varies, of course, according to the iron contents of the soil. The greater amount of the element, stored up as it is in the outer layers and in the germ of the kernel, is lost in the modern milling processes. The organic iron compounds of the germ seem to play an important part in the germination of the seed and in the nutrition of the young plant which not unlike that of the new-born animal, requires easily digestible and assimilable food. Experiments indicate that the iron in bran is also assimilated by the animal body, and promotes the formation of hemoglobin.

Fruits and nuts contain an appreciable amount of iron, strawberries and walnuts ranking highest. Of the vegetables, those bearing greenest leaves always have the largest amount of iron compounds. But we must remember that in order to produce normal food products, special attention must be paid to the soil, which should contain an appreciable amount of iron. Frequent analyses of the soil are, therefore, of great importance.

In eggs the iron is mostly contained in the yolk, while the white contains only traces of it. Meat, as ordinarily eaten, the muscular tissues having been washed free from blood, contains but a comparatively small amount of iron. Fatty tissues are nearly free from iron. The quantity of iron in fat meat is much less than that occurring in lean meat.

The importance of green vegetables, especially prepared in wholesome salads, must, therefore, be particularly emphasized, since we are practically dependent upon the vegetable kingdom for the greater part of iron, which is found in plants in the form of highly organized iron-combining nucleo-albumens.

Manganese

Manganese resembles iron in its physical and chemical properties. In nature manganese accompanies iron everywhere. It is contained in the red blood corpuscles, though in much smaller quantities than is iron, and seems to have a decided influence on the vegetative functions and on the glands in general, enabling them to improve the quality of their secretions. Like iron, manganese is an oxygen carrier from the lungs to the cells.

Traces of this element are found through all the vegetable kingdom, and in considerable quantity in the ash of a few plants, especially in the wood of some trees. Experiments have shown, however, that physiologically manganese cannot act as iron in plants in all instances, although the chemical properties of the elements are similar. Soluble manganese compounds may, on the one hand, be injurious to the chlorophyll, while on the other hand they may exert a beneficial action by stimulating the growth of the plant, especially when these compounds are supplied in a sufficiently high degree of dilution. A Japanese investigator in a field experiment with rice recently observed an increase of one-third of the harvest after adding sulphate of manganese compounds in the soil at the rate of forty pounds per acre. Great care should always be exercised in application of both iron and manganese compounds in the soil, as an over supply of these elements has a detrimental effect on the growth of plants and trees.

Dr. E. V. McCollum has shown that animals deprived of manganese lose the maternal instinct, refuse to suckle their young, do not make a nest for them, and will even eat them. They do not have proper development of the mammary glands, nor do they secrete normal milk for their young.

Foods high in manganese are lettuce, potatoes, wheat germs, almonds, walnuts, peanuts, kelp, dulse and agar. Most fruits and vegetables contain an appreciable amount of it.

ALUMINUM

As Revised By

LILLIAN R. CARQUE,

NATURAL BRANDS RESEARCH FOUNDATION.

Aluminum is the third most abundant metal in known terrestrial matter, including the solid earth, the waters of the earth, and the surrounding atmosphere Oxygen ranks first at 50.02 per cent, silicon 28.50 per cent, aluminum 7.3 per cent, and iron at 4.18 per cent.

As aluminum is widely distributed in Nature, pro-aluminum interests lead us to believe that its presence is to be expected in vegetable and animal tissues, in plants because of its occurrence in the soil, and in animals as derived from plant foods and drinking water. Since, however, the aluminum of the earth is in combination mainly as oxides and silicates, both quite insoluble, *no great concentration can be reached at any one time in the bodies of plants or animals.* That is why aluminum appears in foods in minute quantities, and cannot be separated completely from iron and other metals.

We submit herewith extracts ferreted out of the findings of the Mellon Institute Of Industrial Research, sponsored by the Aluminum Company of America, as contained in their A SELECT, ANNOTATED BIBLIOGRAPHY ON THE HYGIENIC ASPECTS OF ALUMINUM AND ALUMINUM UTENSILS, Bibliographic Series Bulletin No. 3, representing the most authoritative source on the pro-aluminum viewpoint; subsequently to be followed by a brief summary taken from the voluminous data of Dr. Charles T. Betts, author of ALUMINUM POISONING, revealing the recognized position of the opposition:

Mellon Institute Of Industrial Research Point No. 1: On any supposed beneficent influence exerted by the appearance of aluminum or its compounds in the soil:

"In amounts exceeding those which are of value to plant germination and growth, the ions of each of these metals exert toxic action, the toxic action of iron being greater than that of aluminum."

"In highly alkaline soils, toxicity may be dependent on the presence of aluminate ions."

"Aluminum may enter the plant and be translocated, but does not appear to exert a true toxic effect when present as simple ions. Non-toxic aluminum may accumulate in the plant, and appears to render the tissues susceptible to disease."

Mellon Institute of Industrial Research Point No. 2: On Attacks of Aluminum Cooking Vessels on Foods:

"Foods were prepared according to standard recipes "Boston Cooking School Cook Book") in aluminum utensils, with controls prepared in exactly the same manner but in pyrex glass. All of these were then analyzed for their aluminum content. The control analysis gave the aluminum content of the foodstuff, the difference between this and that of the food cooked in aluminum presented the aluminum take-up."

Aluminum Content

Foodstuff	Duration of Cooking Min.	Cooked in Glass p.p.m.	Cooked in Aluminum p.p.m.		Av. Increase in Aluminum p.p.m.
Boiled ham	120	0.78	2.1		1.32
Creamed chicken	120	0.95	2.43		1.39
Percolated coffee	15	0.25	1.03		.78
Oatmeal	150	1.51	9.13		7.24
Stewed tomatoes	20	0.12	4.36	Bright pan	4.16
Stewed tomatoes	20	0.14	15.6	Dark pan	15.3
Sauerkraut	45	0.83	16.4		15.6
Green beans	90	0.91	2.28		1.37
Navy beans	180	1.44	3.60		2.16
Creamed cabbage	45	0.37	2.76	Cooked without soda	2.41
Creamed cabbage	45	0.34	90.8	Cooked with soda	90.5
Cranberry sauce	10	0.53	7.90	Bright pan without sugar	7.36
Cranberry sauce	10	0.63	3.20	Bright pan with sugar	2.54
Cranberry sauce	10	0.52	28.00	Dark pan without sugar	27.5
Cranberry sauce	10	0.75	3.50	Dark pan with sugar	2.70
Rhubarb	5	0.95	13.45	Bright pan	12.5
Rhubarb	5	0.94	41.8	Dark pan	40.9
Apricots	40	24.6	73.3		48.7
Prunes	40	4.60	7.10		2.50
Apple butter	390	5.28	118.00	Includes time to concentrate cider	113.00
Orange marmalade	90	.30	3.06		2.76
Lemon-pie filling	2	0.31	2.24		1.93.

"Metal stirring utensils should be avoided due to the possibility of starting a galvanic current by contact with the walls of the vessels which would promote the solution of aluminum. Therefore to prevent undue corrosion, it is recommended to use wooden spoons for stirring during cooking."

"In a determination of the suitability of various pure metals and alloys for use in the orange products industry, a study of their corrosion rate was made by half submerging metal plates in boiling orange juice for three consecutive 24-hour periods. Of the various metals tested, the aluminum compounds showed the greatest corrosion; from 0.003 to 0.004 inches per month—5 times as great as nickel, 50 times as great as some of the alloys." "In tomato, apple and red grape juices, aluminum was much more resistant than iron and tin, though slightly less so than the other metals used. In lemon juice, however, the resistance of aluminum was poor, the loss exceeding that of tin after 18 hours."

"It was observed by the French during the war that beef preserved in aluminum cans contained from 1-145 mg. of aluminum per 100 g. of material, but that a concentration of over 50 mg. per 100 g. could be detected by a metallic taste. When the preserved beef was stored in aluminum cans for over 1 year, temporary gastrointestinal symptoms resulted in its ingestion."

"Samples of aluminum and various aluminum alloys were exposed to superheated steam at 300° to 350° C. for nine hours daily for 34 days. Pure aluminum showed the most corrodibility, the sample being totally destroyed by the exposure to steam."

Mellon Institute Of Industrial Research Point No. 3: On the Pernicious Influence of Alum (aluminum) Baking Powders:

"When such (baking powders) are used, the amount of aluminum ingested (possibly 250 mg. daily) is much greater than that resulting from the use of aluminum cooking utensils."

"The solubility in the stomach of aluminum compounds found in baking powder residues has been studied in eighteen subjects. With an ingestion of 15 to 90 mg. of aluminum, from 0.4 to 14.6 mg. have been found in the gastric contents in soluble form, comprising from 2 to 20 per cent of the amount ingested."

"Tests carried out on human beings fed with farinaceous food containing alums showed that on an average about 10% of the total aluminum in the food was absorbed by the stomach juices, and there are indications that most of this was reabsorbed into the system in the usual way."

*Mellon Institute Of Industrial Research Point No. 4: On the Allegation that the Use of Aluminum Utensils is provocative of cancer:**

"The absorption of aluminum is so light that there is little danger of toxic effects when taken by mouth in moderate amounts. Both iron and aluminum are of toxicological importance when administered hypodermically."

"The lethal dose of aluminum chloride for rats is from 7 to 8 g. per kg. This dose, given subcutaneously, produced death in 1 to 3 days. The liver and kidneys showed outstanding injury."

"Warm and cold blooded animals are susceptible to large amounts of aluminum when it gets into the blood, causing general paralysis with lowered sensibility, hyperemia and congestion of the gastro-intestinal canal. He concludes that aluminum compounds which go over into the blood may cause poisoning."

"Aluminum is excreted through the gastrointestinal wall, a fact which may explain the difficulty noted in finding it in large amounts in the blood."

"Hospital patients awaiting operation were then given meals containing aluminum, and blood let during the operation was analyzed. Again traces of aluminum were found."

**It is generally conceded that cancer is due to chronic poisoning of the system over a period of twenty to thirty years. Were the body kept up to par by proper diet, thus eliminating constipation, foreign substances might not prove so dangerous. Eminent authorities overwhelmingly sustain the position that malignant growths are caused by a highly toxic condition of the blood. They likewise emphatically urge an early removal of all precarious lesions and sources of chronic irritation.

LILLIAN R. CARQUE.

"The amount (storage) increases with advancing age." "Only very large doses, indeed, have been found to give rise to certain phenomena of physiological irritation."

"It is recognized that soluble aluminum salts, in comparatively large doses are toxic and may tend to produce gastric ulceration in the same way as other *non-specific irritating substances.*" (Italics ours.)

Mellon Institute Of Industrial Research Point No. 5: On Aluminum Attacking Brain and Nerves:

"Most bad effects attributed to aluminum are the result of phosphate starvation due to aluminum phosphate precipitation."**

"The absorbed aluminum circulates in the blood, is stored especially in the liver, ***brain,*** kidneys, spleen and thyroid."

The following brief recapitulation of the findings of Dr. Charles T. Betts, author of ALUMINUM POISONING, with the exception of poisonous degree claimed, is substantiated by some of the conscientious probings of the Mellon Institute of Industrial Research, sponsored by the Aluminum Co. of America.

Dr. Betts Point No. 1: On Attacks of Aluminum Vessels on Foods:

"When ordinary water or foods come in contact with aluminum, the metal, without breaking or chipping, constantly dissolves and becomes part of the food product contained therein. In this form it combines with various chemical elements, like salt, soda, etc. used for seasoning purposes and with the foods themselves. A poisonous substance is produced by such combinations."

"The poisonous effects of aluminum compounds are inimical and as pronounced, whether taken from aluminum cooking utensils, alum baking powders, in drinking water or when prescribed as a medicine."

Dr. Betts Point No. 2: On Aluminum and Cancer:

"Aluminum is not a constituent part of the human body and it is not a necessary element to its proper functioning."

"Aluminum in all its forms, when taken into the body has great activity and has such an absorbing power that an acidosis condition or constipation usually follows its use."

"A normally healthy body can dispose of much of such poison, but when one is subnormal and resorts to medication for bowel action, the aluminum poisons are apt to be reabsorbed into the blood and follow the circulation again. This may become a persistent or habitual operation, causing continual poisoning.

Dr. Betts Point No. 3: On Aluminum Attacking Brain and Nerves:

"Aluminum acts as a general poison upon the brain and nervous system. It has been conceded by the manufacturers of aluminum products that if the residues from prepared foods containing such materials gain access to the blood or are in reality soluble or are absorbable by the body, evil effects to the nervous tissues and other organs would be the result."

Copper

By OTTO CARQUE

Copper has been found in the liver and gall, as well as in the blood. It is also a constituent of some fruits, especially apricots. Although the amount contained in the human body is very small, about 15 grains, copper seems to have a biological significance. In an endeavor to find out just what the substances might be which had value in addition to iron, laboratory workers

**Phosphorus is a natural constituent of the brain and nerves.
LILLIAN R. CARQUE.

in the University of Wisconsin, after test feedings with various substances, and gradually trying various factors of the substance found to be of special value, finally concluded that copper was the significant material. When this decision was made, many investigators quickly confirmed it.

Relation of Copper to Iron

Iron and copper also furnish interesting examples of the nutritional effects of numerous elements. The red color of the blood is due to an iron compound in the hemoglobin. With a diet deficient in iron, the blood becomes pale and anemia results. But one can become anemic on a diet abundant in iron salts—for another metal, copper, must also be present. By its catalytic action, copper helps in the transfer of iron from food to the blood. It is therefore very important that the food shall supply sufficient amounts not only of iron, but also of all other elements and substances which may be needed in connection with the assimilation of iron and its transformation into hemoglobin. Copper has lately been found to function without iron in this connection; and it is held by some investigators that manganese also may in some way facilitate the process of hemoglobin formation.

According to analyses made, the following amounts of copper were found in 1000 grams of the foods named below:

10 kinds of nuts	11.6 milligrams
4 kinds of legumes	9.0 milligrams
19 kinds of cereals	4.7 milligrams
8 kinds of dried fruits	4.2 milligrams
4 kinds of poultry	3.0 milligrams
17 kinds of fish	2.5 milligrams
2 kinds of garden legumes	1.7 milligrams
11 kinds of roots and tubers	1.4 milligrams
14 kinds of leafy vegetables	1.2 milligrams
27 kinds of fresh fruits	1.0 milligrams
10 kinds of non-leafy vegetables	0.7 milligrams

Copper has also been found in appreciable quantities in wheat germs, oats, rye, corn, barley and in asparagus.

Lithium

By OTTO CARQUE

Lithium has been found in very small amounts in all parts of the human body and according to some investigators it is found chiefly in the lungs, and seems to influence the metabolism of the albuminous substance.

Zinc

By OTTO CARQUE

Zinc exists in very minute quantities in connection with phosphorous in the tissues of the brain. It also has been traced in milk and seems to be necessary in the nutrition and growth of certain plants. According to some experiments, zinc is also connected with the action of the vitamins, which it can replace in the animal organism to a certain extent.

Nickel

By OTTO CARQUE

Nickel has been found in very diminutive quantities in different organs of the body, especially in the insulin of the pancreas. Probably nickel is an active ingredient of insulin, which is essential for the proper oxidation of the sugar in the tissues, just as iodine is the active principle in thyroxin of the thyroid gland.

CHAPTER XI

THE ACID-FORMING ELEMENTS

The principal acid forming elements in the body are: phosphorus, sulphur, silicon, chlorine, fluorine and iodine.

Phosphorus

Phosphorus is chiefly found in nature in the form of phosphates of calcium, iron, and aluminum, which minerals form deposits in some localities, but also occur diffused in small quantities through all soils upon which plants will grow, phosphorus being an essential constituent of plant protoplasm.

Phosphorus in the isolated state is manufactured chemically from bones, which contain fifty-eight per cent. phosphate of calcium and four per cent. phosphate of magnesium. The element appears as a colorless, transparent substance which has somewhat the appearance and consistency of bleached wax. In the course of time, and especially upon exposure to the light, it changes by degrees and becomes less and less translucent, gradually turns white, yellow and finally, yellowish-red.

The most characteristic features of phosphorus are its great affinity for oxygen, and its luminosity. It is visible in the dark (phosphoresence), from which property its name, signifying "carrier of light," has been derived. Because of its affinity for oxygen, phosphorus has to be kept under water, as it invariably takes fire when exposed to air. The oxidation takes place upon the surface of the phosphorus, soon raising it to 122° F., at which temperature it ignites and burns with a bright white flame, and gives off dense white fumes of phosphoric dioxide. Phosphorus is insoluble in water, slightly soluble in alcohol, and if brought in contact with living tissues, causes burns. Taken internally it acts as a strong poison.

In the plant, phosphoric acid takes part in the formation of the very complicated compounds of the various forms of lecithin formula and nucleoproteins, which are integral parts of every vegetable and animal cell. Phosphorus enters the animal body chiefly in combinations, and only to a small extent as salts. Phosphorus leaves the body in the same form in which it entered the plant, namely as phosphate. The embryos of plants can develop by cell division only when phosphates are stored up in sufficient quantities in the seeds for the formation and increase of the nuclear substance in the new cells. The yield of grain is increased more by phosphoric acid than by nitrogen or potash.

In the vital processes of the animal, *lecithins,* phosphorus compounds, play a most important part. They have, in common with fats to which they are closely allied in composition, the property of solubility in alcohol and in ether But at the same time they have the power of swelling in water, and even being somewhat soluble in it—a property which renders them physiologically superior to ordinary fats.

Lecithin seems to be essential to respiration, as it represents the form into which the fat must be changed to become oxidized in the protoplasm, since the substances serving for respiration must be present in the protoplasm in a dissolved condition. It is this peculiarity which enables lecithin to take part in many other chemical processes in the tissues. The brain and the nervous system contain an appreciable amount of lecithin, and the gray matter of the brain shows seventeen per cent, of this substance, which is the essential and indispensable basis of the more intelligent animal life.

Phosphorus Does Not Produce Thought

Although phosphorus is one of the principal constituents of the brain, the expression of Moleschott, "no thought without phosphorus," is not justified if it meant to convey the idea that the amount of phosphorus passing through the body bears a casual relation to the intensity of thought. A captive lion or tiger assimilates and parts with a greater amount of phosphorus than does a person performing difficult mental labor, while the excreta of a beaver, noted for its powers of contrivance, are so small that chemical analysis can hardly find it.

The greater the purity in which lecithin is found the higher the intelligence of the animal, even in the smallest insects. The superior acuteness of senses displayed, for instance, by bees and ants, is due to this fact.

It may be asserted that for proper functioning of the brain a supply of phosphoric salts is necessary, but the same may be said with equal justice of oxygen, carbon, water, etc. The intensity of thought does not depend on a single element, but on the perfect working order of brain and nervous system, in which the compounds of phosphorus are essential. But this element itself does not produce thought, any more than do the other elements entering into the composition of brain and nerve cells.

In the organic world phosphorus is generally combined with potassium as phosphate of potash, and as such it makes up the greater part of the mineral contents of the seeds of plants and of the muscular tissues of animals. All the organs and tissues of the animal body are to a considerable extent chemical combinations of phosphates and of proteid matter. The bulk of phosphorus, however, in vertebrate ainmals is contained in the skeleton. In the body of a normal man, weighing about 150 pounds, there are about thirty ounces of phosphorus, of which twenty-seven ounces are in the bones, a little over two and one-half in the muscular tissues and about one-fourth ounce in the brain and nervous system. In cases of prolonged fasting the necessary amount of phosphorus is largely contributed by the bones, while the brain remains almost intact.

The accumulation of phosphorus in the nucleo-proteids of seeds and muscular tissues leads to a conclusion that this element is a powerful stimulant in the growth and development of new tissues, perhaps largely due to its great oxidizing powers. In this respect phosphorus is counter-balanced by sulphur, which plays the part of a regulator, protecting the organism from over-stimulated growth. The relation of phosphorus and sulphur in our foods is, therefore, worthy of careful attention.

Sulphur

Sulphur is found in the elementary state, mixed with earthy matter in volcanic districts, the chief supply being derived from Sicily. Considerable quantities also are mined now in Utah, Nevada and California. In combination sulphur is widely diffused in the form of sulphates and sulphides. Sulphur is a yellow, brittle, solid substance, having neither taste nor odor. It is insoluble in water and nearly so in alcohol. It melts at 239° F. and if heated to 500° F., burns with a blue flame to sulphur dioxide.

In the organic world sulphur is built in the proteid molecule of the plant from the sulphates taken from the soil. It is chiefly taken up by the animal organism in the form of protein, and secreted for the most part in the highest oxidized condition as sulphuric acid, derived from the splitting up and oxidation of the protein molecule. In this form, combined and neutralized by alkalies, it is again ready to begin the cycle of life, by forming organic sulphur compounds in plants.

Sulphur is a constituent of the hemoglobin of the blood, where it also serves as an oxidizing agent. It is noteworthy that, according to analyses, the animals requiring more oxygen have likewise more sulphur in their hemoglobin. Four atoms of sulphur in the hemoglobin of the horse, six in that of the dog and nine in that of the chicken, go to two atoms of iron. Sulphur enters into the composition of albumen, gelatin, etc., in all of the tissues. It is one of those elements that make up the natural resisting power of the body, as the organized sulphuric acid salts have a cleansing and antiseptic influence in the alimentary canal.

The Relation of Phosphorus to Sulphur in Nutrition

All organic building material contains phosphorus and sulphur at the same time, although in very different proportions. The phosphates (the combinations of phosphoric acid with the basic or alkaline elements) serve pre-eminently for the purpose of giving the actual impulse to growth. This is explained by the fact that we find phosphate of potash in all seeds and germs which have to give birth to new organisms. The seed that is put into the soil has, above all things, to grow as rapidly as possible, so that it can reach out in both directions, to send its tiny roots downward and its small stems and leaves upward that they may absorb further nourishment from earth and air. Seeds, in order to give the embryo plant every chance for growth, contain therefore, comparatively little sulphur. Likewise, in the animal body those parts which are intimately connected with growth show a marked preponderance of phosphorus over sulphur. Thus we find that the skeleton contains a large amount of phosphate of lime and of magnesia, the muscular tissues, phosphate potash, and the brain and nervous system, lecithin. While in the blood the proportion of sulphur to phosphorus is 1 to 2, it is in the muscular tissues and brain about 1 to 65.

Many diseases of the nervous system are due chiefly to the unbalanced proportion in which the elements of sulphur and phosphorus are supplied in the usual foods (principally cereals and meat). Such conditions as mental irritability, neurasthenia, abnormal sexual desires, insanity, etc., are very much aggravated by an excessive amount of phosphoric acid. Furthermore, an oversupply of phosphorus and nitrogen in our diet, with a simultaneous deficiency of sulphur and sodium, lead to abnormal tissue formations such as polypi, tumors, elephantiasis, cancerous growths, etc. There are many pathological conditions which may appear to the uninformed physician as being entirely heterogenous, but which really have the same source, namely: an insufficient supply of sulphur, sodium and of calcium, with a preponderance of phosphorus, potassium and of nitrogen foods. For instance, obesity, asthma, rheumatism and hemorrhoids are many times merely different symptoms of one cause—the inadequate supply of sulphur, iron and of calcium. These elements supplied in natural foods are the essential basis of normal albumen of the blood or hemoglobin. On the condition of the latter depends the capacity for absorption of oxygen in the system, and consequently, perfect oxidation.

Many diseases, which hitherto have been ascribed solely to the accumulation of uric acid in the system, are really caused by the consumption of foods which are too rich in phosphoric acid and deficient in sulphur. This is the case with all foods which abound in nucleo-proteins, although they contain but very little uric acid, such as milk, cheese, eggs, nuts and cereals. These foods should never be taken as an exclusive diet, but always in small quantities properly balanced with fruit and vegetables rich in sulphur to counteract the excessive amount of phosphoric acid salts.

Considering the nutrition of man in the light of above facts, we find explanation for many diseases which arise from faulty metabolism—diseases which are hardly noticed in the beginning but which become more firmly established in the course of years; and then years of the strictest hygienic living and self-denial are required to eradicate, or at least to alleviate them. The excessive use of white flour products in occidental countries as the fundamental cause of abnormal formation of tissues, of cancerous and nervous diseases, asthma, obesity, diabetes, etc. finds its correlative in the more or less exclusive fish and rice diet of the oriental countries, as the source of leprosy, beri-beri, etc. Almost every civilized nation has its characteristic diseases, arising from faulty nutrition and living. Thus we find gout and rheumatism predominant among the meat-eating Northern peoples, while pellagra is found in the Southern European countries, chiefly in Italy, where people live on macaroni, maize, cheese and wine. While macaroni, maize, cheese, rice and fish are not injurious in themselves, it is their demineralized forms and injudicious use that is the source of mischief.

The polaric distribution of sulphur in plants should also be considered. During their growth this element is carried to the stem, leaves and skins of fruits and of seeds, corresponding to the accumulation of sulphur in the skins, sinews, hair and in the feathers of the animal body. Nature here follows a definite object. Sulphur, like silicon, has a good insulating power which holds the electricity of the body together, preventing its premature and too rapid dissipation, and at the same time giving all those parts of the body containing it, softness, elasticity and pliability.

Silicon

Silicon, or Silicium, is found in nature very abundantly as silicon dioxide or silica in the form of rock-crystal, quartz, agate, sand, etc. It exists also in the form of silicates, which are silicic acid in which the hydrogen has been replaced by metals. In most of our common rocks, such as granite, porphyry, basalt, feldspar, mica, etc., are such silicates or a mixture of them. Small quantities of silica are found in spring waters, as well as in vegetable and animal substances. In the organic world silica is most effective as a protective agent against chemical disintegration and putrefaction. The element has, therefore, a strong antiseptic action, being a safeguard against epidemic diseases. The mineral matter from healthy muscular tissues contains at least two per cent silica, which is also found to a considerable extent in hair, feathers, nails and in claws. In vegetable foods the silica is combined with cellulose, and forms the skin of fruits and vegetables and the outer coats of cereals. In white flour, also corn meal, polished rice, etc., this coat has been removed in the form of bran. This deficiency of silica gives rise to many diseased conditions and makes the system easily susceptible to injurious influences. Silica, being a good insulator, warms the blood by insulating and by keeping together the electricity imparted by its salty constituents. Silicon is found most particularly in the connective tissues. As nerve substance contains nearly the same amount of silica as does the albumen in the blood, this element forms, as it were, a connecting link between blood and nerves, preserving their proper relations. Many diseases of the blood and nervous system are aggravated by a lack of silica in the food.

The pancreas is especially rich in this element, its mineral constituents showing about twelve per cent of silica. It is found combined with fluorine in the enamel of the teeth. Human hair shows from 0.10 to 0.23 per cent. The hair needs for its growth silica and sulphur. If these are not supplied in sufficient quantities to the blood, the hair cannot be nourished properly and falls out. The skin, and likewise the walls of all cells, contain a considerable amount of silica, which has been placed there by nature to prevent a too rapid radiation of the body's heat and electricity. We, therefore, see that silicon, like the other elements, has certain physiological functions to perform, which makes its presence in our food and, consequently, in the different parts and organs, indispensable. The amount of silicon in the body may be small as compared with other elements, but its importance as an essential building element of the body should never be overlooked. The rapid spreading of so-called infectious diseases must largely be accentuated by a deficiency of this element in the system, as the average diet of man usually lacks silica. The ash, for instance, of the outer coats of the rice kernel contains almost eighty per cent of silica, which is to a large extent lost by the peeling, and further by the polishing process. In the same manner silica is lost in the artificial preparation of all cereal foods. In peeling fruit we also lose an appreciable amount of organic salts. Wherever it is possible, fruits should be eaten with the skin, which must, of course, be properly masticated.

Chlorine

Chlorine is found chiefly in sodium chloride or common salt, either dissolved in water (small quantities in almost all spring water, larger quantities in some mineral waters, and the greatest amount in sea-water), or as solid deposits in the interior of the earth as rock-salt. It may be isolated by chemical processes when it appears as a yellowish-green gas, having a disagreeable taste and an extremely penetrating and suffocating odor, acting energetically upon the air passages, producing violent coughing and inflammation. Chlorine is about two and one-half times heavier than air and is soluble in water. There are but few elements which have as strong an affinity for other elements as has chlorine. The act of combination between chlorine and other elements is frequently attended by the evolution of so much heat, that light is produced, or in other words, combustion takes place.

In the vegetable kingdom chlorine occurs mostly in the form of potassium chloride and of sodium chloride. Small quantities of sodium chloride applied to the soil have a beneficial action on various crops, and to an extent increase their resistance to drought and to rust fungi. When the amount of sodium chloride reaches a certain degree of concentration in the soil, however, injurious effects will be observed. A solution of 1.8 per cent sodium chloride will prevent the germination of wheat. The assimilation process in the leaves is also retarded by a surplus of sodium chloride in the soil. Other injurious effects are the decrease of sugar in the sugar beet, and of starch in the potato. An over-supply of potassium and of magnesium chlorides also depresses the starch content of the potato.

Chlorine, in the form of sodium chloride, plays an important part in the animal organism. It asists in the formation of all the digestive juices, principally of the gastric juice, which contains two per mille hydro-chloride acid. The mineral matter of the blood serum is largely made up of sodium chloride which favors and sustains the generation and conduction of electric currents. About one-third of the ash of the white of hen's eggs consists of sodium chloride. Milk also contains a large amount of chlorine, which perhaps may be explained by the fact that the chlorides are useful, not only in the construction of the organs but also in the preparation of the digestive secretions.

Chlorides are likewise important for renal secretion. They are necessary for the elimination of the nitrogenous waste products of metabolism. This is shown by the fact, among others, that diuretics also increase the excretion of chlorine. The fact that sodium chloride is a normal constituent of the human body, being present to the extent of 6.5 per mille in the blood, has given it special importance in the eyes of the people, and has lent credence to many exaggerated popular notions regarding its curative effects. Whenever the inorganic salt is ingested, it draws fluid from the tissues rapidly and there results an increased discharge of urine, greatly exceeding the quantity of water ingested. This produces the sensation of thirst which leads to the excessive imbibing of liquids and of consequent weakening of the kidneys. The inorganic coarse salt also diminishes the secretion of hydrochloric acid, it causes peptones to become deficient. and disturbs the absorption of sugar.

Fluorine

Fluorine exists chiefly in nature as fluorspar and as calcium fluoride. Traces of fluorine occur in many minerals, in some waters, and also in the bones of mammals and in the enamel of the teeth. Fluorine was until 1887 scarcely known in the elementary state, because all attempts to isolate it were frustrated by the powerful affinities which this element possesses, and which renders it difficult to obtain any material for the manufacture of a vessel which is not chemically acted upon, and therefore destroyed by flourine.

Fluorine exists in small quantities in nearly all plants and animals. It is chiefly found as fluoride of calcium in the bones and teeth of men and of mammals, but the exact amount has not yet been ascertained. Fluorine has also been detected in the blood of birds and of mammals, as well as in the yolk of eggs and in milk, where it is chiefly combined with fat, also in the outer coats of grains.

Fluorine is necessary for the formation of the enamel of the teeth, and is needed in the development of the skeleton, as no normal bony substance can be formed without fluorine. The iris of the eye, which reflects the whole organism, also requires fluorine. A deficiency of the element in the lens of the iris is followed by opthalmic diseases. The artificial preparation of our food stuffs by which the greater part of the fluoride of calcium is removed or made inert, also the inadequate supply of this substance to the soil is one of the principal causes of premature decay of the teeth, curvature of the spine, and of early weakening of the eyesight.

A deficiency of calcium fluoride causes a lack of elastic fiber or rubbery material in muscular tissue. "Elastic fiber is formed by the union of the fluoride of lime with albuminoids, whether in the rubber tree or the human body" is indicated on page 30 of THE ZODIAC AND THE SALTS OF SALVATION. In other words, the threads or filaments are incapable of expanding and contracting, resulting in a prolapsed uterus, with very painful and weakening female troubles following in its wake; varicose veins; flat foot due to a relaxed condition of the elastic muscular fibers or connective tendons which hold the arch in place. An insufficient supply of calcium fluoride also causes rupture or hernia and a general sagging down feeling mentally as well as physically.

Iodine

Iodine is a non-metallic element, found in small quantities in many plants and animals. In its free state the element is soluble in ether and in alcohol, but only slightly so in water.

The element is present in the thyroid gland to the extent of about two per mille. of the dried weight of the gland or about ten or fifteen milligrams (¼ grain) in the entire gland. It is essential for the formation of an organic iodine compound—thyroxin—which regulates some of the metabolic functions of the organism. A lack of iodine prevents the formation of thyrosin and causes enlargement of the thyroid gland or goitre. This disease is common in certain districts of the European Alps and of the Rocky Mountains. It is probably caused by an insufficient and one-sided diet, and by a lack of iodine in the soil. As sea-water contains iodine, it is naturally present in all sea plants, such as algae, kelp, Irish moss, dulse (sea lettuce), etc.

According to Dr. Bourcet, a French chemist, iodine occurs in the following products of the vegetable kingdom. The amount is given in one-millionth parts of fresh substance.

Pineapple	0.310	Tomatoes	0.023
Green kidney beans	0.320	Pears	0.017
Asparagus	0.240	Artichokes	0.014
Cabbage	0.210	Dry white beans	0.014
Garlic	0.210	Lettuce	0.012
Mushrooms	0.172	Grapes	0.010
Strawberries	0.170	Potatoes	0.010
Whole rice	0.134	Oat flour	0.009
Leeks	0.120	Whole wheat flour	0.007
Sorrel	0.120	White flour	0.000
Green peas	0.080		

All salt water animals, as well as salt water plants contain an appreciable amount of iodine, as sea-water contains potassium iodide and sodium iodide.

Of 18 analyses of milk none showed iodine; cereals, especially, if deprived of their outer coats, are practically devoid of iodine, while non-starchy vegetables seem to contain a comparatively large amount of this element. In regions where a large amount of dairy products and of cereal foods are eaten and not enough of the fresh vegetables and fruits, especially where the soil is deficient in iodine, goitre seems to be prevalent.

When the iodine in the thyroid has been used up and it can no longer supply the needed secretion to the system, various body functions begin to be affected. The part the thyroid secretion (which really means iodine) plays in the lives of humans, is admirably summarized by Dr. Barwise, an English Medical Officer, in an official report made by him in 1924:

"1. It is necessary for effective metabolism, and specially promotes respiratory exchanges and physical growth.

"2. It promotes efficient mental development. A severe shortage before birth results in cretinism. An inadequate supply may produce anything from imbecility to mere mental dullness.

"3. It is especially required in the pregnant condition, and antenatal clinics must bear this point in mind.

"4. It is needed at the age of adolescence for the development of the reproductive organs, particularly in the female, in whom the changeover takes place more rapidly than it does in the male.

"5. It is needed to keep the skin and its appendages in a healthy condition. A dry skin and falling hair frequently mean a thyroid deficiency.

"6. It is required for the digestion, assimilation and combustion of fats. When a shortage occurs the fats cannot be satisfactorily dealt with, and it is stored in the subcutaneous tissues. Many cases of obesity may be occasioned in this way.

"7. It is required for the metabolism of calcium.

"8. It is needed to enable us to resist the invasion of microbes, and to render harmless the toxins (poisons) they produce."

Arsenic

Arsenic, which occurs in the earth as sulphide of arsenic, is found in minute traces in animals and in vegetables. Until recently it has not been considered essential to their well-being. The French chemist Bertrand, however, as a result of numerous experiments, has arrived at the conclusion that arsenic, instead of being a constituent of a few tissues only, is a constant element of the living cell. He finds arsenic present in the eggs of all fowls, in exceedingly small quantities, the yolks generally containing twice as much as do the whites.

In 1900 Dr. Gautier, of Paris, established the fact that arsenic in a very small proportion enters into the constitution of the outer tissues, of the epidermis, hair, nails, thyroid gland, brain and of the breast. There are some traces of it, but much less, in a few other organs. Arsenic appears to resemble in its chemical affinities those of phosphorus.

Bromine

Bromine has been found in the liver, thyroid gland, adrenal glands and in the nails. It has not been definitely established what physiological functions this element performs. In the vegetable kingdom bromine occurs chiefly in sea-plants (algae, etc.).

CHAPTER XII

THE VITAMINS

Much has been written of late about vitamins. Many books have been published about their supposed properties, and scientific researches have been made to establish their identity. Whatever the final results of these controversies may be, they have brought about some important readjustments in the theories of nutrition. By numerous laboratory experiments in feeding animals on all the isolated food principles, such as proteins with the essential amino acids, carbohydrates, fats and mineral matter, (in the proportions in which they were supposed to be necessary for complete nutrition), it was found that after a few days the animals lost weight almost as rapidly as if they had been starved. As soon as they were given natural food, such as milk, however, in which all the constituents are compounded into an organic whole by the great universal life force, they began to put on weight again. Thus the fact was clearly established that, while animals can live on milk alone, yet if all the proximate principles of milk, which according to the present teaching of physiology are necessary for the maintenance of the organism, are artificially mixed together, the animals rapidly die.

The same holds true in regard to all natural foods, whether fruits, nuts, vegetables or cereals. We cannot deprive these foods of certain parts or of certain organic combinations, without at once depreciating their nutritive value. There must, therefore, be something in nature's products which we cannot imitate, and which we may call the life principle, the same mysterious force which develops a seed into a plant, a beautiful flower, a lofty tree, an insect or a man.

Vitamins are intimately connected with the building of the protoplasm itself. Their supposed functions have been likened to those of electric sparks in the forming of new organic combinations essential to growth. The author is inclined to believe that vitamins are integral parts of protoplasm, resembling the amino acids in their composition and that their vital action largely depends on certain organic salts in the cell which act as catalysts. No electro-vital and chemical action in the cell can take place without the necessary mineral elements. It is futile, therefore, to discuss the action of vitamins independently from the physiological functions of the organic salts.

One of the scientists who devoted considerable time to the study of this problem is Dr. Casimir Funk. He named these elusive substances of the organic world *vitamins*. This name is derived from the Latin words *vita*, meaning life, and amins or amino acids, which are component parts of the protoplasm The subject was further investigated by Drs. Osborne and Mendel, of Yale University, and by Drs. McCollum and Davis, of John Hopkins University.

It seems that during the last ten years the science of nutrition has paid too much attention to the vitamin question, neglecting other important biological factors. No matter how important vitamins may be, we cannot live on them alone, any more than we can on any one of the other proximate food principles. It is very probable that the different vitamins have special relations to other food ingredients, such as iodine, fluorine, calcium, iron, phosphorus, etc., and that only in organic combination with these elements can they exert their beneficial influence. In other words, any proximate food principle must be chemically united with the other constituents into an organic whole, such as we find in the form of wholesome natural foods.** As has been already stated, whatever may be claimed for the vitamins, their chemical and biological actions must always be studied in close connection with those of the organic salts and of amino acids, if we want to come closer to the solution of the problem of rational nutrition.

The vitamins whose functions have been determined are the following:

Vitamin A

Fat Soluble Vitamin "A" or *anti-opthalmic vitamin* seems to occur mostly in the green leaves of plants, such as spinach, lettuce, cabbage, alfalfa, clover, etc., in tomatoes, carrots, sweet potatoes, yellow corn, green peas, etc.; also in butter-fat, egg yolk, palm oil, cod liver oil, in liver and kidney tissues and in the glandular organs in general. The solids of spinach and tomatoes contain more of vitamin "A" than does butter-fat. The latter, as it exists in milk, is essential to the normal growth of the child, or the young of animals, and a deficiency ot it will produce stunted growth, emaciation and rachitic conditions.

In many animals, as rats, dogs, rabbits, and poultry, and also in man, a characteristic affliction of the eyes results, known as ophthalmia, or xerophthalmia. This is such a characteristic and almost universal consequence of Vitamin "A" deficiency that it is regarded as a specific disease. The administration of Vitamin "A" prevents and promptly alleviates this disease. Growing animals require more Vitamin "A" than do adults. In man, a condition of impaired vision called "night blindness" is known, particularly in Arctic regions. During the recent World War and following it, many children in Europe suffered from an eye affection, which was readily relieved by the administration of cod liver oil, which supplied the Vitamin "A".

The separation of butterfat from milk removes most of the Vitamin "A" from milk. Butter, cream, and cheese made from whole milk are therefore

**Research Laboratories have succeeded in isolating vitamins as independent organic structures. Vitamin D, for example, is a separate fat soluble entity, and occurs only as fat is present. Vitamin D does help the organism to utilize advantageously the available calcium and phosphorus, serving as it does as a regulator or economizer of these minerals. None the less, there is no fat in di-calcium phosphate and only two to three per cent in vegetable leaves. Thus it may be seen that calcium-phosphorus compounds, as bone ash or as these elements occur in plant or mineral life, have no relationship to Vitamin D.

LILLIAN R. CARQUE

very good sources of Vitamin "A". The commercial condensing, evaporating and drying of milk does not appreciably reduce its content of this vitamin. Cereals, as a class, are not good sources of this vitamin. Oats, rice, wheat, barley and white corn contain but little, if any of it. It is definitely associated in some way with the pigments of plants, and is found in significant quantities in yellow corn, Japanese millet, and in haricot beans. Green peas have been recently reported to be an unusually rich source of Vitamin "A". It is generally present in fruits.

It has been demonstrated that the Vitamin "A" content of milk varies directly with the vitamin content of the ration of the cow. Milk richest in this vitamin is obtained from cows feeding on pasturage. Stall-fed cows in winter, living largely on cereals, dry feeds and cured hay produce milk that is relatively low in Vitamin "A".

Vitamin B

Water Soluble Vitamin "B" is contained principally in plant foods, the seeds of cereals, when not impoverished by modern milling processes, peas, beans and in other legumes in their natural state, as well as in yeast, milk, roots and tubers. Citrus fruits furnish a considerable amount of vitamin "B", more than do the deciduous fruits. Nuts contain a considerable quantity, and, like vitamin "A", it is also found in the green-leaf vegetables. An insufficient supply of the vitamin "B" as for instance in a diet largely of peeled or polished rice, results often in a specific nervous disease known as beri-beri. In order to maintain health in young and old, a constant supply of "B" is required. Anti-neuritic Vitamin B-1 is a substance necessary for the normal growth of the animal and human organism, for the maintenance of appetite, and for the adequate tone, mobility, and functioning of the stomach and intestines, large and small.

Lately it has been found that Vitamin "B" consisted of more than one factor; one factor which was affected by heat, and another one which was heat resistant. At one time Dr. Sherman proposed the use of the term Vitamin F for the anti-neuritic factor now recognized as B-1; and B-2 is now designated as Vitamin G for the factor which has been found to prevent pellagra.

Vitamin C

Water Soluble Vitamin "C" is supposed to be present in large amounts in fresh fruits; to a less extent in raw vegetables and tubers; in moderate quantities in milk and meat. Among fruits the best sources are oranges and lemons: among the vegetables, various turnips, carrots, rhubarb and tomatoes. Baked potatoes also contain moderate quantities. An absence or insufficient supply of vitamin "C" produces scurvy.

Vitamin "C" is the least stable of all the vitamins. It has been estimated that ordinary kitchen cooking may destroy from one-half to three-fourths or more of the Vitamin "C" originally present in the raw product. Acid products, as tomatoes and fruits, can be cooked with but little destruction of Vitamin "C". The effect upon the vitamin content of foods caused by the process of dehydration varies both with the method used in drying and also with the nature of the particular fruit or vegetable. Dried fruits retain a considerable part of the vitamin "B" and but little or none of Vitamin "C".* Acid fruit juices, as orange and lemon juice, can be desiccated with little or no loss of vitamins. Some vegetables, on dehydration, lose most of their Vitamin "C" content, particularly cabbage and turnips. Storage at low temperature has but little effect on Vitamins "A" and "B", while it destroys Vitamin "C" to some extent. By pasteurizing milk, Vitamin "C" is agitated and aeration results. Sterilization under similar conditions destroys it completely.

Vitamin D

Fat Soluble Vitamin "D" controls the metabolism of calcium and phosphorus in bone-building and teeth-formation. It prevents rickets, poor development of teeth and faulty metabolism of calcium in the body. It is found principally in cod liver oil, and to some extent in butter fat. This vitamin may aptly be called the "Sunshine Vitamin" according to the experiments made by Professor Steenbock of the University of Wisconsin, who showed that the amount of Vitamin "D" in foods can be increased by exposing them to ultra-violet rays, a process which is called "irradiation."

With a series of brilliant experiments, Professor Steenbock worked out the fact that rickets can be prevented in animals in several very remarkable ways. The most direct way is by letting the animals themselves make their Vitamin "D" in their skins by absorbing the rays of the ultra-violet light. But he also found that the animals could get their sunshine second-hand by drinking the milk of goats which had been similarly exposed to ultra-violet rays.

The distinctive thing that Professor Steenbock has done is to prove that this creation of Vitamin "D" is not exclusively a function of the rays of the sun acting on a live animal, but the same action can also be secured in the foods themselves. The substance that is changed by sunlight to Vitamin "D" is called *ergosterol* or *viosterol,* the latter name given to it because it is a vitamin developed from sterol of plant origin.

In young animals the administration of cod liver oil or irradiated ergosterol, or direct ultra-violet irradiation, has been shown by many investigators to raise the level of blood calcium and phosphates to relieve tetany and to heal rachitic lesions.

**It is only fair to say that there is a greater conservation of Vitamin C in sulphured sun-dried fruits. The sulphuring process seals the pores of the fruit in a manner that does not permit a more thorough evaporation. Hence there is a higher moisture-retention content in the flesh of sulphured fruit, as compared with that in sulphur-free dried fruit, which makes possible swifter processing. Vitamin C in unsulphured fruits is thus destroyed through too long exposure and oxidation, but this inadequacy can be remedied admirably by the continued and persistent consumption of citrus fruit abounding in this vitamin.

LILLIAN R. CARQUE

The adult who wishes to keep his Vitamin "D" balance at high level may use irradiated foods, or he may produce his Vitamin "D" by getting plenty of sunlight, taking sunbaths whenever possible.

The reason why cod liver oil contains Vitamin "D" is because there are on the surface of the ocean trillions of tiny creatures called animalcules or plankton (chiefly protozoans) who constantly absorb the ultra-violet rays of the sun. These floating microscopic creatures of light are eaten by the small fish, which in turn serve as food for the larger fish whose liver provides a storehouse for Vitamin "D". Thus sunlight is carried to the sunless depths of the sea in the body of the big cod. However, we do not have to get our vitamins in this round-about fashion from the liver of the cod. Green-leaf vegetables that grew in properly fertilized soil and that were fully exposed to sunlight, are the natural, best and most economical source of all the vitamins, especially if these vegetables are eaten as nearly as possible in their natural state.

Vitamin E

Fat Soluble Vitamin "E" also called ***anti-sterility vitamin,*** was originally referred to as Vitamin "X", because of the uncertainty, due to lack of knowledge about it, as to whether or not it should be classed as a vitamin. Most of the knowledge concerning this vitamin has been obtained within the last few years. It has been shown that rats reared on synthetic food mixtures containing fat, carbohydrate, protein, salts, and Vitamins "A" and "B", grow well and have every appearance of health, but exhibit complete sterility, affecting both males and females. In the case of the male, eventual destruction of the germ cells resulted. In the case of the female, however, although the ovary and ovulation remained unimpaired, a characteristic disturbance occurs in gestation, involving the death and reabsorption of the developing young. When small quantities of natural food stuff were added to the ration of these same rats, there resulted in many cases, normal-sized litters of vigorous young.

The richest source yet found of Vitamin "E" is the germ of the wheat kernel. It is also found in oats and corn. Green leaves also contain this vitamin—lettuce, alfalfa, tea and peas. Its occurrence in cottonsed oil and in commercial olive oil, but not in coconut oil, linseed oil or in sesame oil, has been reported. It is present, but never highly concentrated, in animal tissues, being higher in the musculature and fat than it is in the viscera. Milk contains it in extremely small quantities and cod liver oil is notably lacking in this vitamin.

Vitamin "E" is soluble in ether, and it shows remarkable stability as compared with other vitamins. It can withstand strong acids and alkalies and high temperatures.

An excess of Vitamin "E" cannot increase fertility beyond normal limits.

Vitamins F and G

Vitamin "G" (B2) was discovered not so much by any special investigation as by a gradual growth of evidence, which finally became fully convincing. It supporting the common assumption of identity between "antineuritic vitamins" was shown by experiments that not all of the evidence could be considered as and "water soluble 'B' " (regarded as a growth-promoting substance). As already stated, Vitamin "B" comprises a complex of the anti-neuritic vitamin, and of a more heat-stable part, to which the term vitamin G (B2) has been applied.

Cereals, legumes and probably all seeds, are relatively less rich in Vitamin "G" than in Vitamin "B". By experiments made at the University of Illinois, it was found that twice as high a proportion of the ground whole grain in a food mixture was needed to meet the Vitamin "G", as to meet the Vitamin "B" requirement.

It has been found that Vitamin "G" is essential to the growth of young rats; and here is abundant proof that it is likewise necessary for the growth of mammals and man.

Foods which show an appreciable amount of Vitamin "G" are:

Apples
Asparagus
Avocado
Bananas
Beet roots and leaves
Buttermilk
Cabbage
Carrots
Cauliflower
Cream
Watercress
Eggs
Grapefruit
Lettuce
Oranges
Fresh peas
Pears
Potatoes
Salmon, canned
Spinach
Tomatoes
Turnips
Wheat germ
Milk
Milk, skim
Milk, evaporated
Yeast

Vitamin "G" appears to be formed principally in the growth of the green plant; and according to investigations at the Ohio Agricultural Experiment Station, there are indications that the amount of Vitamin "G" in the leaves and succulent stems may decrease as they dry and wither.

As vitamin "C" is most easily affected by heating, a liberal amount of fresh fruit and vegetables, therefore, is always necessary to maintain health. Sufficient quantities of Vitamin "A" may be obtained from cooked, or better still steamed vegetables, retaining their juices. "B" occupies an intermediate position. and while raw cereals, which contain this vitamin, cannot be recommended as ideal food for man, they should always be used in their natural form, such as whole rice, whole barley, whole wheat bread, whole corn meal, etc.

The vitamins, whatever their chemical composition may be, must be active in extremely minute quantities, and in that respect, they resemble the enzymes in their catalytic actions, producing chemical changes without undergoing any change whatever in themselves. The vitamins, however, seem to be most actively engaged in the building and reconstructive processes of the organic cell, within which sphere the ultimate processes of nutrition take place.

We may admit that Vitamins are indispensable to the process of nutrition and of growth in the vegetable and animal kingdoms. Equally important, however, are the mineral elements or organic salts in our food, especially in their relation to each other in the normal growth of the body, in the performance of the various physiological functions of the organism, and last but not least, in the preservation of its health and in the power of resistance to injurious influences.

NEW VITAMIN FINDINGS

As Supplemented by
LILLIAN R. CARQUE, Director,
NATURAL BRANDS RESEARCH FOUNDATION

Vitamin F

The following data is taken from a treatise entitled VITAMINS AND MINERALS by Arthur W. Snyder, Ph. D.:

"The name Vitamin F has been given to certain unsaturated fatty acids; these unsaturates are found in butter, lard, linseed oil and some vegetable oils. They are also found in the human skin in small amounts.

"The function of Vitamin F in human nutrition has not been definitely established. It is credited with helping to maintain the proper resilience and lubrication of all cells. Vitamin F seems to be of distinct benefit to the skin, nails and hair. It has been used with considerable success in bronchial asthma, hay fever and allergic eczema.

"Deficiency of Vitamin F may cause dry skin, weak dry hair, brittle finger nails, baldness, acne, eczema, dandruff, distress in hot weather, and allergic conditions. Vitamin F has been extensively used in cosmetics and hair preparations. No official unit has yet been established."

VITAMIN H

Again we quote from VITAMINS & MINERALS by Dr. Snyder:

"Vitamin H is an acid substance found in yeast, liver and kidney; in rats a deficiency of this Vitamin causes psoriasis and a form of eczema. Research is being carried on to determine its value to humans."

VITAMIN I

The following is extracted from the PHYSICIANS' VITAMIN REFERENCE BOOK edited by the Medical Division, Professional Service Department of E. R. Squibb & Sons, New York:

"Vitamin I: An anti-infective (possibly anti-pneumoccic) factor which, it is alleged, is present in lemon juice."

Vitamin K

The data hereunder is again taken from the Squibb PHYSICIANS' VITAMIN REFERENCE BOOK:

"Nothing is known as yet about the human requirements for Vitamin K. Apparently most individuals on balanced diets obtain enough through the diet, but when there is obstruction of the bile duct so that bile is excluded from the intestine, evidence indicates that Vitamin K is not absorbed.

"SOURCES: Green leafy vegetables, such as spinach, alfalfa and cabbage are excellent sources of Vitamin K. Tomatoes, hog liver and hempseed are also good sources.

"Vitamin K is known as the 'coagulation' factor because it appears to be necessary for the formation of prothrombin (necessary for the first step in the process resulting in formation of a blood clot). It is being tried clinically for the prevention of prolonged hemorrhage in the treatment of various forms of jaundice and in pre-operative and post-operative treatment of patients with obstructive jaundice.

"Snell reports separately on a patient with obstructive jaundice due to stricture of the common bile duct, and with a badly damaged liver and virtually incoagulable blood. Normal coagulation followed administration of a diet rich in Vitamin K.

"A curative method of assay has recently been developed by Ansbacher (Squibb Institute for Medical Research). It is based upon the observation that the clotting time of the blood of Vitamin K-deficient chicks becomes normal within a very short time after the administration of Vitamin K. His unit is defined as that amount of vitamin which is necessary to reduce the clotting tme of the blood of the K-deficient chicks to normal within six hours after administration.

"Vitamin K is fat-soluble; it is non-nitrogenous; contains an aromatic nucleus; does not contain phosphorus or sulphur; can be distilled in a high vacuum; is not particularly stable; apparently does not contain a sterol ring; is alkalilabile but fairly heat-stable. A melting point of 60° C. is reported for the crystalline substance."

Synthetic Vitamin K has been too recently introduced to permit comment.

VITAMIN P

The following is again taken from VITAMINS & MINERALS by Dr. Snyder:

"Vitamin P, also called the flavone factor and citrin; is a factor of Vitamin C in lemon juice. It helps to strengthen the capillary walls and tends to prevent hemorrhages. Acts on the capillaries tending to bring back their resistance and also alters the permeability (penetrability) of the capillaries and for this reason was assigned the letter P. By helping to prevent the passage of serum proteins through the capillary walls into tissues, Vitamin P has proved helpful in edema or dropsy."

From the Squibb PHYSICIANS' VITAMIN REFERENCE BOOK we note:

"Vitamin P: This is claimed to be a factor responsible for certain hemorrhagic symptoms of experimental scurvy in guinea-pigs.

"Citrin: Another name for Vitamin P."

VITAMIN T

Again we quote from Squibb's PHYSICIANS' VITAMIN REFERENCE BOOK:

"Schiff and Hirschberger (Berlin) reported the presence of a principle in sesame oil, but not in cod liver oil or olive oil, which produced thrombocytosis (blood clot) in children. This work has not been confirmed."

Dr. Casimir Funk on Vitamins

By OTTO CARQUE

Dr. Casimir Funk, who first investigated the nature of the vitamins, when once interviewed, expressed the opinion that the American public would do well to curb its tendency towards making a fad of artificially supplying vitamins in various preparations. He said in part:

"What would be the use in preparing all our foods artificially, so long as nature is producing her own foods in sufficient abundance to supply an increasing population? It would be folly even to think of turning ourselves into domestic manufacturers and consumers of self-made food so long as nature gives us enough."**

In regard to milk Dr. Funk said:

"The contents of vitamins in milk have been greatly exaggerated. There are other foods that are far richer in vitamin content than is milk. We are by no means dependent upon milk alone for our supply of vitamins.

"The vitamin content in both mother's and cow's milk is essential for infants. But vitamins are not any magical possession of either milk. They exist there because the mother or the cow has assembled them from the food she has eaten prior to the production of the milk."

It is evident that the quality of mother's milk, or that of any animal depends largely upon the quality of food consumed. If the food is impoverished, naturally the milk cannot supply the necessary elements for growth. Cow's milk should not be used without knowing how the animals are fed and cared for.

Nature's Distribution of Vitamins

By OTTO CARQUE

Foods which contain all five vitamins are: alfalfa, germinating seeds, fresh clover, lettuce and sea vegetation (kelp and dulse).

Foods containing vitamins "A", "B", "C" and 'D" are bananas, string beans, buttermilk, raw cabbage, carrots, carrot juice, green onions, grapes, kohlrabi, lemons, raw milk, oranges, orange juice, grapefruit, raw spinach, raw and canned tomatoes, turnips.

Foods especially rich in Vitamin "C" are apples, peaches, pears, grapefruit, lemons, oranges, raspberries, lettuce, parsley, fresh pineapple, strawberries, tomatoes, turnips, bean sprouts, cucumber, watercress, peppers and germinated cereals. If fresh vegetables or fruit are scarce or absent, an anti-scorbutic food can be prepared by moistening any available seeds (wheat, barley, rye, peas,

**While Nature does give us enough food, it is idle to deny that as fast as the soil is being depleted, so chemically deficient have our foods become. Hence the imperative need for satisfactory nutritional adjuncts, grown on properly fertilized soil, to supplement even a natural and rational dietary.

LILLIAN R. CARQUE

beans, lentils, soy beans) and by allowing them to germinate or sprout. It is necessary, of course, that these should be in the natural whole condition, not milled or split. The seeds should be soaked in water for 24 hours and kept moist with access to air for one to three days, by which time they will have sprouted. This sprouted material possesses an anti-scorbutic value equal to that of many fresh vegetables. They should be cooked for as short a time as possible.

Products entirely deficient in vitamins are: polished rice, soda crackers, tapioca, starch, refined sugar and hydrogenated oils, unless irradiated or fortified with added vitamin concentrates. Margarine contains only a trace of Vitamin "A", if unfortified.

Sunlight and Irradiation

By OTTO CARQUE

Experiments have shown that sunlight is effective in curing and preventing rickets. Sunlight is in effect a substitute for Vitamin "D". Animals on a diet containing no Vitamin "D" quickly develop rickets when kept in the dark, but when exposed to direct sunlight rickets does not develop. The ultra-violet rays in sunlight are responsible for this action. These rays do not pass through window glass, so that direct exposure to sunlight is essential for this effect. If cod liver oil is added to the rickets-producing diet, however, normal development follows even in comparative absence of light. Among the most remarkable recent discoveries is the fact that many substances, having naturally no antirachitic properties, as cottonseed oil, olive oil, linseed oil, lettuce and spinach, can be made highly active by irradiation with ultra-violet rays. Green lettuce leaves from the market have little value in preventing rickets, whereas after irradiation they acquire antirachitic properties. Milk exposed for two hours to ultra-violet light has been reported to be effective in curing children severely afflicted with rickets. Cholesterol, a compound found in animal tissues, contains normally no Vitamin "D", but after exposure to ultra-violet light it is rendered antirachitic. Even more remarkable are recent results obtained showing that when out of a colony of rachitic rats in the same cage, one was taken out and irradiated and then placed in the cage with the others, the irradiated rat not only improved, but even imparted to the rachitic animals the beneficial effect of the irradiation.

VITAMIN PREPARATIONS

By OTTO CARQUE

In the green leaf of the plant we find all the material necessary for the preservation of life. While vitamin preparations contain only one or more of the vitamins (invariably more than one) we find in the green parts of vegetables many of these substances contained in a highly active state and in favorable quantities. The same is also the case with the mineral constituents of which I have made a study. Most all artificial food preparations exhibit the same peculiarity with regard to minerals as to vitamins—there is always a superabundance of one constituent or another, or else some are absent altogether or are present in too insufficient a quantity. Furthermore, it must be understood that the maintenance of health and development does not depend solely on the total number of mineral substances present, but largely on the proportion of these substances to one another, particularly on the ratio between acid carriers and the basic mineral substances. *All these obligatory conditions are fulfilled by green leaves.*

Consequently, *all artificial preparations are more or less unbalanced,* simply because the fundamental knowledge necessary for their manufacture is entirely lacking. *Only living plants can give us all the factors necessary for the maintenance of health.***

VITAMIN CONCENTRATES EXPLAINED

Supplemented by

LILLIAN R. CARQUE

NATURAL BRANDS RESEARCH FOUNDATION

Since the late Otto Carque's passing, it has become possible to extract the various vitamins from their natural sources, or to prepare synthetic chemical substances believed to possess human biological values identical with certain of the vitamins. Many vitamins have been isolated as pure substances, each with its own definite chemical formula and structure, and artificial synthesis of some has been definitely accomplished.

Ethical vitamin preparations represent the quintessence or highest potencies of various food concentrations known to abound in one or more specific vitamins. For example, highly potent preparations of Vitamins A and D may be prepared from fish liver oils. Vitamin A, per se, is not synthesized from the structures of various forms of plant life. Its precursor, provitamin A or carotene (often highly condensed from fresh carrots or high-grade alfalfa) is, however, readily converted or manufactured into Vitamin A itself when ingested by human and animal organisms.

Thiamin Chloride (synthetic Vitamin B-1) is generally acknowledged to be as effective for its specific purpose as is Vitamin B which occurs in Nature. The organic compound Thiamin or its salt Thiamin Chloride can be synthesized just as any known organic substance can be synthesized. It has none the less been

**Synthetic vitamin and mineral preparations must of necessity be unbalanced for remedial purposes. We are all more or less unbalanced or incorrectly polarized, often with exaggerated mental, moral and psychic conditions; hence there is a definite predominant need of one or more kinds of vitamins and minerals to restore equilibrium.

Some evidence in better medical literature and practice indicates that clinically recognizable single vitamin deficiency diseases are rare in this country. None the less, partial or latent deficiencies are relatively common but no less potentially serious, for a deficiency disease is seldom limited to only one factor. In the presence of multiple deficiency, the use of preparations containing a combination of vitamins offers the obvious advantage of simplicity of administration for both the physician and the patient. Such combinations may also be more economical than the equivalent dosage of the vitamins obtained by the use of separate preparations.

LILLIAN R. CARQUE

claimed that ascorbic acid (synthetic Vitamin C), also called cevitamic acid, does not contain all the antiscorbutic (scurvy-preventing) properties found in such citrus fruits as oranges and lemons. While synthetic Vitamin C has not given uniformly parallel results to the vitamin from the natural source, it proves very satisfactory in the treatment of scurvy, and as a prophylactic measure when citrus fruit juices are refused or are tolerated poorly, and where there is a pathologic interference with the assimilation of the amount of Vitamin C necessary to preserve health.

Low ascorbic acid levels have been noted in patients with gastric and duodenal ulcers, also with ulcerative colitis due to an intolerance of citrus fruits in their prescribed diets. Clinical evidence reports rapid response to massive doses of synthetic Vitamin C in relation to the healing of peptic ulcers. Hence it seems reasonable to add supplementary vitamins, especially ascorbic acid (synthetic Vitamin C) to the usually approved ulcer regimens. In patients with whooping cough, the University of Manitoba (Canada) reports that administration of the synthetic Vitamin C shortened the paroxysmal stage from weeks to days. Improvement in the general condition was rapid and noticeable.

Vitamin D occurs only as fat is present. It is known to be associated with fat soluble entities indicated as sterols. Exposure to ultraviolet light of these various fat substances produces energies with varying Vitamin D potencies. It is recognized that there are two major sources of Vitamin D; animal and vegetable. The source of animal origin refers to those forms presumably related to cholesterol, as found in fish liver oils or irradiated milk. The plant sterol (ergosterol), when irradiated or activated by solar energy, produces a substance which is commercially designated as "Viosterol."

Evidence has appeared in the literature which suggests strongly the superiority of animal source Vitamin D in respect to the inhibition of dental decay in humans. One of the earliest studies on the relation of Vitamin D to dental decay —that of M. Mellanby in England (British Medical Research Council)—showed that a relatively large dosage of Viosterol gave poorer protection against dental decay than did a relatively small dosage of cod liver oil.

Vitamin E is obtained from several concentrations of the sperm of various seeds; the most economical source is wheat, in the form of cold-pressed wheat germ oil. The various factors of Vitamin B complex (Vitamin G or B^2) may be obtained in concentrated form from the natural sources of wheat germ or rice polishings. The recognized organic substance in Vitamin G is considered to be riboflavin, and the pellagra-preventive property of the B complex is understood to be nicotinic acid.

It is obviously most desirable for individuals to obtain their full share of the various protective food factors—vitamins and minerals—as a part of their normal diet. Yet it must be considered that fortified foods and concentrates do afford an additional source of important dietary essentials needed for the attainment of optimal nutrition. Certain high potency vitamin preparations have their place in human nutrition because many factors in modern living tend to affect, adversely, the natural vitamin value of the ordinary diet. These may be due to soil deficiencies; to loss of vitamins in commercial processing and refining; to economic conditions responsible for malnutrition; to faulty preparation of food for the table and unhygienic dietetic habits; and finally, because of a frequent need for high dosage in concentrated form to overcome more or less severe vitamin deficiencies arising from numerous physical conditions which limit the assimilation of the vitamins from the digestive tract, or which interfere with storage through vomiting, diarrhea, etc. "It is becoming more apparent that prolonged inadequacy of vitamins, either from dietary lack, failure or utilization, or increased demand (in the organism) produces a variety of borderline states of ill health," say Doctors Williams and Spies in their treatise VITAMIN B_1 AND ITS USE IN MEDICINE.

CHAPTER XIII

RATIONAL SOIL FERTILIZATION

What has been said about mineral elements, in their relation to the rational nutrition and normal growth of the animal and human body, may to a large extent be applied to the vegetable kingdom. Plants and trees often suffer from a deficiency or excess of certain elements in the soil. These conditions naturally cause poor crops and lowered stability of the plant protoplasm, making it susceptible to rapid disintegration and to the attack of fungi and insects. We should, therefore, recognize the fact that the soil must contain all the essential elements for the growth and propagation of plant life in an assimilable form and in the right proportions in order to bring forth wholesome and durable products, which in turn are necessary for the normal development of animals and man. Man will always be dependent on the soil, whether directly or indirectly, for his sustenance, but we can never expect to build healthy, strong and enduring bodies from foods grown on impoverished or wrongly fertilized soil.

Modern agricultural chemistry dates back about sixty years, when the late Baron Justus von Liebig published his work, "Natural Laws of Husbandry," in which he said:

> "No intelligent man who contemplates the state of agriculture with an unbiased mind, can remain in doubt, even for a moment, as to the state of husbandry in Europe. We find that all countries and regions of the earth, where man has omitted to restore to the land the conditions of its continued fertiliy, after having attained the culminating period of the greatest density of population, fall into a state of barrenness and desolation. Historians are wont to attribute the decay of nations to political events and social causes. These may, indeed, have greatly contributed to the result; but we may well ask whether some far deeper cause, not so easily recognized by historians, has not produced the downfall of nations, and whether most of the exterminating wars between different races may not have sprung from the inexorable law of self-preservation. It may seem to the superficial observer that nations, like men, pass from youth to age, and then die; but if we look at the matter a little more closely, we shall find that as the elements for the continuance of the human race which nature has placed in the soil are very limited and readily exhausted, the nations that have disappeared from the earth have dug their own graves by not knowing how to preserve and renew these materials. Nations (like China and Japan) which know how to preserve the fertility of their soils have not died out.
>
> "Not the fertility of the earth, but the duration of that fertility, lies wihin the power of the human will."

While Liebig recognized the injurious effect of an excessive supply of nitrogen in the soil, in the form of guano, nitrates, stable manure, he still believed that a liberal supply of potash and phosphoric acid was most essential for plant growth. He drew this conclusion from the analysis of grain, without taking into account the stems and leaves, which especially require lime, iron and magnesia for their growth and development.

Boussingault's Defective Experiment

The theory that nitrogen must be the essential element of all fertilizers, and that it must be applied to the soil because the plant can not take it up directly from the air, was chiefly propagated by the French chemist, J. B. Boussingault. The misleading experiment from which he drew the conclusion that plants are incapable of absorbing and using atmospheric nitrogen impressed the agricultural chemists of his day as an indisputable demonstration of the truth of his ideas.

We know now that leguminous plants are capable of obtaining from the air all the nitrogen they need, and while we find no nitrogen in the roots and trunks of forest trees, their leaves contain appreciable amounts of it in the chlorophyll, which is formed by the absorption of nitrogen directly from the air.

We must, therefore, recognize the ability of all plants, not only the legumes, to draw from the air and soil the nitrogen they require without the necessity of an extra supply of this element in the shape of commercial fertilizers. Vast sums are annually spent for various nitrogen compounds with no other result than the production of rankness in early growth, like that produced by means of a hotbed. The leaves and stalks become weak because, during the brief time of their abnormal and rapid growth, they cannot absorb from the soil a sufficient amount of such substances as silicic acid, iron and lime. These are the elements which give to the plant the necessary firmness and power of resistance against injurious atmospheric influences and insect pests. Insects do not propagate very well on leaves and fruits rich in lime and iron, while the stalks of plants, stimulated in their growth by an excess of nitrogen, fail to acquire the necessary stiffness and strength and are always liable to be laid by heavy wind and rain.

Today thousands of farmers who do not have the remotest conception of the real effect of manures upon their crops apply to their land guano, nitrates and other fertilizers, for which they pay many millions of dollars. All this waste of money is due to Boussingault's defective experiment, which is still accepted as conclusive evidence by most of the agricultural writers and teachers.

Boussingault set about his famous experiment in the following way: He grew seeds in sterilized pumice stone, adding a definite quantity of certain minerals needed for the plants. He then arranged to supply water, carbonic acid and nitrogen from the air through an ingenious system of tubes, causing the air containing nitrogen to pass through sulphuric acid, so as to free it of any ammonia it might contain. The experiment was carried on under a glass globe.

After the plants had grown to maturity chemical analysis showed that the amount of nitrogen was exactly the same as had been contained in the seeds, from which they were grown. Apparently the plants had not absorbed any nitrogen. Boussingault proclaimed this as an absolute proof that plants are not able to absorb atmospheric nitrogen and form it into plant protoplasm, but must draw all the nitrogen they need from the soil.

Boussingault, however, overlooked the fact that the growth of plants inside the glass globe released so much oxygen that any atmospheric nitrogen was prevented from entering the globe. The theory of the absolute necessity of nitrogen fertilization was, therefore, derived from two misleading circumstances: first, there was no way for the oxygen released by the plants to escape from the globe, and second, no nitrogen could enter the globe.

It has also been proven, that wherever marly limestone is present in the soil or is applied to it, a vigorous growth of vegetation follows without the application of any nitrogen fertilizer. This is explained by the fact that moist carbonate of lime has a strong affinity for nitrogen, which unites with hydrogen and oxygen by the agency of lime to first form nitric acid, and then nitrate of lime. As the sap of all plants contains some iron and lime in solution, there are two ways by which atmospheric nitrogen may be taken up, when water is evaporated from the leaves. A bulletin issued by the Ohio State Experiment Station at Wooster shows that a plot of land given no nitrogen yielded better returns than the plot which received the full amount of nitrogen, as advised by the followers of Boussingault.

Nevertheless, the manufacturers of commercial fertilizers have propagated the idea that the use of phosphoric acid, potash and nitrogen was the only way out of our dilemna of greater production or of starvation. On the other hand, the idea of permanent soil building on a foundation of lime combined with soil humus, whether derived from stable or green manures has been woefully neglected by the vast majority of land owners; it has only recently been forcing itself to the front among the more intelligent agriculturists. The liberal application of animal manure alone may produce large crops, but they are of inferior quality. Manure is an unbalanced plant food, supplying too much nitrogen and not enough of the basic mineral elements; it is especially deficient in lime. The continuous application of manures produces acidity of the soil which should be corrected by the addition of carbonate of lime or marl to the manure, before it is used as fertilizer.

Lime is not only of value as a corrector of soil acidity but as a most essential plant food. It takes part in plant growth, but when deficient, the plant lacks hardiness and is unable to withstand unfavorable cultural and climatic conditions. Lime accumulates mainly in the leaves and stems of plants, where it plays a most important part in the production of new tissue. The mere production of fruit does not draw too heavily on the lime supply of the soil, but in the growth of trees upon which fruit is produced, there is a much larger demand for lime. Fruit trees and vines contain almost 100 pounds of lime carbonate to the ton of wood, and all plants contain a larger or smaller quantity of lime. This means that the quality and flavor of fruit, the size and health of plants are all affected by the supply of lime in the soil. The use of lime on lands well supplied with humus secures for the farmer, without additional cost, all the otherwise expensive nitrogen his crop needs.

Carbonate of lime is the necessary compound for the formation of starch in the growth of vegetables and fruits and cannot be replaced in this important function by any other substance. Lime is essential in the collodial structure of the fruit cells. Fruits grown on soil rich in carbonate of lime are sweeter, more delicious and have a better shipping quality than have those grown on soil treated only with manure or nitrogen fertilizers. Vegetables grown on limed soil keep fresh and crisp, while those forced by stable manure soon wilt after they are gathered.

The Importance of Mineral Fertilizers Proven by Practical Experience

There is absolutely no doubt that all plants, not only legumes, are able to obtain some of the required nitrogen from the air, and a further supply from the earth, if there is sufficient iron and carbonate of lime in the soil. The free use of nitrogen fertilizer is not only useless, but harmful to plants and animals. The effect of nitrogen fertilization on cereals leads to a bright green color growth of soft, sappy tissue with thin cell walls, which are easily attacked by insect and fungoid pests. Liberal application of nitrogen to a field of clover will make it appear luxuriantly green and heavy. But this is deceptive, for a closer examination will reveal that the stalks and leaves are soft and tender, and entirely lacking in the elements that give strength and durability. Truck gardeners may prefer to use nitrates; they improve the outward appearance of such leaf crops as cabbage, lettuce, spinach, etc., and make them, therefore, more salable. But such products do not stand handling and decay rapidly. Soft and flabby tissues, whether in plants or animals, are the result of a deficiency in the essential mineral elements, and such vegetables are unfit as food for animals and man. The injurious effect of nitrogen fertilizers is often increased by the addition of soluble phosphates which hasten the growth of garden truck and small fruit, but destroy the wholesomeness of these most essential foods.

The German scientist, Dr. Julius Hensel, was one of the first to point out the mistakes made in modern agriculture. Like so many pioneers, he was denounced and ridiculed in the most shameful manner by his orthodox colleagues, but Hensel's fundamental ideas of soil fertilization are becoming more and more recognized by all progressive thinkers. In Germany and England an increasing number of farmers are successfully experimenting with his methods of soil culture. When the early agricultural chemists established their theories of manuring with the mineral constituents of the seeds with their high contents of phosphorus, potash and nitrogen, they did not consider that the entire growing plant requires quite different proportions of elements than those found in the seeds alone. Hensel clearly understood what some day all the world will recognize, namely, that plants require a well-proportioned quantity of all the necessary mineral elements for their healthy growth, just as much as man and animals do; that insufficiently or wrongly nourished plants, like animals, fall a prey to diseased conditions more quickly than those specimens which are well built, as a result of an adequate supply of the essential mineral elements.

The late Dr. H. Lindlahr, one of the pioneers of nature cure in the United States, gave the following interesting and instructive data:

"In our institutions for the healing of the sick we begin the treatment of patients by treating the soil of our gardens and farmlands with mineral fertilizers. For many seasons now we have saturated the land with wood ash, sifted coal ash, finely pulverized lime rock, pulverized phosphate rock and iron filings with small quantities of rock-salt.

"The effect of this continued, systematic, mineral fertilizing on the products of our gardens has been little short of marvelous. Every season our vegetable gardens excite the admiration of those who have the pleasure of seeing them."

It is but natural that the manufacturers of the usual commercial fertilizers, containing a surplus of nitrogen and phosphates, strenuously oppose all new ideas of sensible soil culture and condemn all mineral fertilizers as worthless and fraudulent. It is a pity that most of the commercial fertilizers are highly endorsed by agricultural teachers, who still consider an abundance of nitrogen the most essential factor in ascertaining the value of any fertilizing material. In fact, laws have been enacted to prohibit the sale of any substance for fertilization which does not come up to the required nitrogen contents.

Dr. Louis Berman says in his interesting book *"Food and Character"*:

"Climate must be considered as working in combination with soil chemistry. In Tennessee, new-born colts, calves, and other animals reared where the soil is rich in mineral elements like iron, iodine, manganese, copper, and cobalt, are much stronger and more vital than those raised in other regions. Analysis of fruits and vegetables from a mineral-rich region shows them to be quite different from samples grown in other parts of the country. The amount of iodine in oranges, or iron in spinach, for example, may be quite different, depending upon where they have been grown. Wheat grown in the blue-grass districts of Kentucky contains almost three times as much phosphorus as that cultivated in Wisconsin, Michigan, or Minnesota. The amount of cobalt is quite variable in different regions and soils. Cereals, fruits, and vegetables vary correspondingly in their cobalt, which occurs in largest quantity in certain limestone regions. According to Weston, the live-stock born and bred in the cobalt-rich limestone country have extraordinarily fine physiques and superior general development. Foods ought to be certified as to soil origin and chemical composition.

"The great Liebig attempted to work out what might be called a *psycho-chemical interpretation* of history based on the conception of exhaustion of the soil by successive exploitation over a period of generations. Exportation of food from a locality would aggravate this exhaustion. The idea is serviceable in explaining the rise and fall of certain great nations, such as the Greek city-republics and the Roman Empire. Nitrogen and phosphorus were what specially concerned him and his interest and propaganda led to the great development of the agricultural fertilizer industry in Germany. Modern research on the variability of the mineral content of different soils tends to confirm his ideas. But a truly adequate psycho-chemical theory of history would found itself upon a summation of the effects of climatic physics and soil and food chemistry as they affect the ductless glands of different peoples and nations."

All those who are further interested in this subject should read Jack Gaerity's valuable booklet, "Bread and Roses from Stones," which deals with the advantages of mineral fertilizers in a concise and interesting way.

The Future of Our Food Supply

Wrong fertilization, which is exhausting the necessary mineral elements out of the soil, is probably the cause of many failures in fruit crops and of more diseased conditions in man and animals than is generally admitted. For years mankind has accepted the idea that fertilization must be done with manure, reinforced with nitrates and phosphates. But it will eventually be found that despite all such fertilization, the land is slowly but surely losing its productiveness; that insect pests increase, and, what is worse, that the quality of the soil's products is deteriorating. Intelligent soil culture will, therefore, be one of the most important problems with which the growing population of the earth will have to deal, for the health and welfare of nations depend in no insignificant measure on rational nutrition.

Investigations along these lines are of such vital importance that the government of every civilized country should take up the extensive study of the subject. The United States Department of Agriculture has made a large number of analyses of food products, but the specific study of the mineral elements and their relation to one another in the healthy growth of plants and animals has been neglected. All nations are spending vast sums for the constant increase of armies and navies and for instruments of destruction. If they devoted but a hundredth part of this money to the advance of agricultural chemistry and to the science of nutrition, it would lessen the need for territorial conquests, and more amiable relations between the nations would result.

Only a short time ago, in an address to the Williamstown Institute of Politics, Rear Admiral Ledyard Rodgers made the following startling remarks:

> "I do not suppose the United States will ever desire to make war against any country before our continental population passes 200,000,000, but after that, if there remains any manhood in our mixed race of descendants, they will assuredly do so to keep their place in the world."

This has been the reasoning of all the militarists, since the time of Alexander, Caesar and Napoleon. The World War, from whose effects our superficial civilization is still suffering, was largely the outcome of our insane system of rapid commercial expansion, exciting the rivalry of individuals and of nations. Everything is raised and manufactured for big profits, regardless of quality, and new markets have to be constantly conquered.

By intelligent and intensive culture of the soil and utilizing all the natural resources in an economical way, the United States can easily supply at least twenty times its present population, giving health and happiness to all, without making war on neighboring countries.

CHAPTER XIV

CLASSIFICATION AND DESCRIPTION OF FOODS

Fruit, Man's Best Food

Rich in Natural Sugars and Alkaline Elements

In the fruit of the tree, nature has produced one of her masterpieces. She has provided an ideal food for the human race. Like man himself, fruit trees appeared late in the order of evolution on this planet. The fact that most of our flower-bearing plants and fruit trees are unknown in a fossil state clearly prove their recent origin which in all probability was synchronous with that of man.

Fruits, which nature develops more slowly than other products of the soil, receive for a longer time the beneficial influence of light, heat and air, through which the electric and magnetic forces of the sun are transmitted. In fruits, therefore, we find the highest manifestation of electro-vital energy and cell vibration of all foods; and while we cannot determine by chemical analysis this subtle quality, we can feel its wholesome and enlivening effects through our whole system. Under the continuous influence of the sun's rays, the elements of the soil, together with water and air, build up the millions of wonderful tiny fruit cells in which all the nourishing constitutents are brought into the most perfect and soluble form. In the ripening of the fruit the sun has taken the place of the cook and produced a morsel of exquisite flavor and wholesomeness, most agreeable to the unpreverted taste and meeting every demand of the body.

The majority of people still regard fruits not as true foods, but merely as accessories to the more concentrated part of their diet. It is this mistaken idea that has lead to an excessive consumption of meat, cereals and dairy products, which overload the system with toxins and overburden the eliminative organs.

The sugar in fruits, combined with organic salts and vitamins, is the body's great sources of potential energy; it is easily assimilated, and enhances our health and endurance. Furthermore, in the process of digestion, ripe fruits—provided they are eaten by themselves and not added to a heavy meal—require only a small expenditure of nerve force. They are more economical physiologically than are starch-bearing and heavy protein foods which, in being assimilated, draw more heavily on our nerve force, and thus overtax and gradually weaken the internal organs, especially the liver and kidneys.

Fruit Sugar
The Most Economical Source of Heat and Energy

Scientific experiments have proved that fruit sugar is the most economical source of animal heat and energy; but one must always discriminate between sugar as it exists in fruits or succulent plants, and the refined sugar of commerce, or that occurring in glucose made from corn starch. Although their chemical composition is similar, fruit sugar is intimately associated with alkaline elements, while refined sugar is absolutely deficient in organic salts; hence while the latter may act temporarily as a stimulant during exertion, it cannot, except for a very brief period, maintain the life processes of the body. When refined sugar is taken, the body cells are rapidly broken down to furnish the blood with the necessary alkaline elements to neutralize the carbonic acid, resulting from the oxidation of the carbon.

The objection has been made that a fruit diet does not supply enough protein. But when we consider the fact that mother's milk at the end of the sixth month of nursing, the time of rapid growth of the infantile body, shows only 1.07 per cent protein, we are justified in saying that fruits, supplemented with very few other foods, which have a higher percentage of protein and some fat, such as nuts or nut butters, or if necessary some dairy products, will give us ample nourishment. Fruits keep the alkalinity of the blood in normal condition, while the more concentrated foods, like cereals, pulses, cheese and meat, are more or less acid-forming. The alkaline elements, which are chemically combined with the different fruit acids, act as natural laxatives by promoting the secretions of the glands. They are also indispensable in preserving the normal physical condition of the epithelium cells, upon which the regular peristaltic movement of the intestines depends.

Moreover, the water contained in fruits is in an absolutely pure state, distilled in nature's laboratory, and is therefore of great value in solving and removing the impurities from the body. In localities where the drinking water is polluted, fruit and fruit juices are well nigh indispensable. Some persons believe that the eating of fruits in the hot countries induces fever. But in most instances the affliction can be traced back to some other cause than that of the partaking of wholesome and natural food.

Fruits may be more expensive than are cereals, as far as their content of solid nourishment is concerned, but the money spent on fruit is a good investment and will return to us ample dividends by increasing our health and vitality. If fresh fruits are not available, dried fruits should be used. The average amount of carbohydrates, mainly sugar, in dried fruits is about 62 per cent; in bread, only 50 per cent.

The principal sweet fruits are dates, figs, raisins and most of the tropical fruits; the sub-acid fruits are apples, apricots, blackberries, blueberries, raspberries, cherries, grapes, peaches, persimmons, plums, and nearly all deciduous fruits. The acid fruits include oranges, lemons, grapefruit, limes, pineapple, pomegranates, strawberries, loganberries, cranberries, loquats, and tamarinds.

Sulphured and Unsulphured Fruits

While dried fruits are not equal in hygienic value to that of fresh fruits, they are the best substitutes for them. They are preferable to canned fruits, containing syrup made from refined sugar or candied fruits. Dried fruits make an ideal breakfast food, especially during winter and spring. They should be used instead of cereal breakfast foods.

In the temperate zone where the season for fresh fruits is comparatively short, a large portion of each crop is now dried, either in the sun where climatic conditions are favorable, as in certain parts of California, or in dehydrators by means of hot air currents. The process of dehydration, if carried on scientifically, is to be preferred to that of sun-drying, for it involves less expenditure of time, and does not expose the fruit to dust and insects.

In the preparation of dried apricots, peaches, pears, nectarines and apples, the fruit is subjected, after the removal of the pit or core, to the fumes of burning sulphur, in what is known as a "sulphur box." This is done for the following reasons:

(1) To produce as clear and intense a yellow color as is possible.

(2) To conceal decayed portions of the fruit which have been overlooked in trimming.**

(3) To prevent fermentation and decay during the drying of the fruit.

(4) To protect the fruit from flies and other insects, the larvae of which would otherwise develop after the fruit was stored.

(5) To make the texture of the fruit less porous; thus higher moisture retention expedites processing.

Fruits which have been sulphured before drying have a lighter color than have those which are dried without sulphuring. At the same time, it is well known that highly sulphured fruits are preserved with a larger percentage of water than are those not subjected to sulphur treatment, and for this reason a greater weight of fruit is produced from a given weight of the raw material when sulphur is used. This is especially the case when the dried fruits are reprocessed in the packing houses. Here the fruits are washed and re-sulphured, increasing the sulphur content of the finished product often to 3,000 parts per million and more.

Extensive experiments conducted by the late Dr. H. W. Wiley, former chief chemist of the United States Department of Agriculture, have shown that the use of a large amount of sulphurous acid in food is always deleterious; that it never adds anything to the flavor and quality of the fruit, but it does render it less palatable and wholesome. Sulphurous acid interferes with the function of the kidneys, which are called upon to remove the additional sulphur from the body. It also retards the formation of the red blood corpuscles.

**In a statement on the "Functions & Effect of Sulphur Dioxide in Dried Fruits," by Dwight K. Grady, it was emphasized that sulphur dioxide is not used for the purpose of concealing inferiority, nor as an adulterant.

LILLIAN R. CARQUE

Although drying or dehydrating fruits greatly reduces their vitamin "C" content in comparison with that occurring in sulphured dried fruits, which seem to retain most of the Vitamin "C", there is one important disadvantage in the use of sulphured fruits. The sulphur dioxide reduces or destroys their alkalinity, according to the amount of sulphur applied. The heavily sulphured fruits of commerce have, therefore, diminished hygienic value.

Here is a reply from the late Dr. Wiley, champion of the Pure Food Law, to whom this question was submitted:

January 14, 1930

"I have no doubt that the gentle acidity produced by sulphur dioxide may help retain the activity of the vitamins in dried fruit, but the way in which the dried fruits are saturated with sulphur dioxide, and especially resaturated at the time of packing, must of necessity injure health to a very considerable degree. The question, then, is whether or not the benefit to health occasioned by the slight increase of vitality of the vitamins is equal to the injury done by the vast quantity of sulphur dioxide used. My own view is that it is better to get our vitamins in some other way than through dried fruits as they are produced at the time. We have plenty of vitamins anyway in our fresh fruits and in our ordinary foods, and do not need this additional amount for the preservation of our health."

Yours truly,
(signed) H. W. Wiley.

Food Inspection Decision No. 76 of the United States Department of Agriculture states that the total amount of sulphur dioxide in the finished product must not exceed 350 parts per million. But much of the sulphured dried fruit marketed in this country carries much more than 1000 parts of sulphur dioxide per million. Certain European countries, France, for instance, have begun to enforce a maximum of 1000 parts per million. In Hungary, Germany and Czecho-Slovakia, 1250 parts per million, in England 2000, and in Canada 2500 parts per million are the legal maximum. New York has named 2000 parts per million as maximum, and New Hampshire has recently prohibited sulphur dioxide in any amount whatever. Most of the states, however, have accepted the federal requirement indicated in Food Inspection Decision 89, issued in 1908, that "ordinary" quantities of sulphur dioxide, if stated on the label, are not objectionable. The objection to excessive sulphuring appears now to be rather on the score of the possible marketing of excessively watery dried fruits rather than that based on the danger of physiological injury resulting from their ingestion.

The author knows from long years of experience in the production of dried fruits, that it is posible by modern processes of dehydration. employing hot air currents not exceeding 120° F., to turn out fairly good-looking unsulphured fruits retaining a good deal of their natural color and flavor. Any deficiency of Vitamin "C" can be supplied easily by fresh fruits and green-leaf vegetables, such as are available now during all seasons of the year, as well as tomatoes, fresh or canned or the addition of some lemon juice. This is the best solution of this problem for those who object even to a small content of sulphurous acid in dried fruits. The sun-drying of unsulphured apricots, peaches and pears requires too long an exposure of the fruit to the air, with the possibility of a slight fermentation and much oxidation and discoloration in case of cloudy weather.

Tropical and Sub-Tropical Fruits

With our improved methods of preserving, transporting and distributing food products, many of the tropical fruits and nuts are rapidly coming within the reach of a large proportion of the inhabitants of the temperate zone. In fact, such products as the pineapple, banana, date and cocoanut have become staple foods in many parts of Europe and of North America. Some of the tropical fruits, hitherto unknown or neglected outside their native countries, are now receiving attention not only in the markets of the temperate zone, but also among growers in subtropical regions, where some of the more hardy varieties of these fruits are being planted. Among the latter, the avocado, or alligator pear may be mentioned.

The *banana* is a striking example of what can be done with tropical fruits, if methods of harvesting, transportation and distribution are improved. The *avocado,* the most conspicuous aspirant for popular favor at the present time, is now grown in a large number of varieties outside of the tropics, hundreds of acres being planted in Florida and Southern California. The avocado equals the *olive* in the amount of fat and protein, but it is more palatable as it can be enjoyed in its natural state. The olive has a bitter taste, which has to be removed by artificial means. However, sun-dried ripe olives, which have lost some of their bitterness, are used by many people in combination with sweet dried fruit or bread. Some varieties of the avocado show a fat content as high as 29 per cent, protein 2.43 per cent, while the total amount of organic salts is much greater than that found in many other fresh fruits. Potassium, sodium, calcium and magnesium compose more than one-half of the total mineral matter. The avocado has a consistency not unlike that of butter. It is richer in protein that are most fruits, while the fat is very palatable and digestible, and much superior to any animal fat. Indeed, this fruit replaces meat to a very large extent in all countries where it can be grown abundantly, as in Mexico and Central America. It is an excellent addition to combination salads, for it supplies both protein and fat, which are more or less lacking in vegetables.

The *orange,* the most important of our citrus or sub-tropical fruits, is one of nature's medicinal foods because of its large calcium and iron content and also its vitamins, "B" and "C." Fresh, sweet orange juice is an excellent food for children to supplement cow's milk. Although the orange contains over 1 per cent of citric acid, the juice, on account of its large amount of potash, is decidedly alkaline in its reactions. Ripe oranges contain as much as 10 per cent of fruit sugar, which is ready for immediate assimilation.

The *lemon,* like the orange, is rich in alkaline elements and has as much as 7 per cent of citric acid. Lemon juice should always take the place of vinegar in the preparation of vegetables salads. The *grapefruit,* or pomelo, less aciduous than is the lemon, is enjoyed by many as a breakfast fruit, especially when sweetened with a little honey. Citrus fruits can now be had in the United States and Canada almost all the year around.

Figs, both fresh and dried, especially Black Mission figs, if free from chemical preservatives, are most wholesome and nutritious for children as well as for adults, and should be eaten instead of candy and starchy foods. The black fig particularly is rich in bone-building elements. It preserves the teeth, is easily digested, and prevents constipation. In its dried state it can now be obtained at all times of the year and should be used freely in every household.

Dates and raisins and many other dried fruits have now become staple foods in all civilized countries and supply our needs when fresh fruits are scarce. Dates and raisins contain about 70 per cent of natural sugars in an easily assimilable form.

Amount of Fruit Consumed in the United States

Although the fruit market in the United States has been greatly extended by improved methods of transportation and storage, the per capita consumption of fruits of all kinds is surprisingly low. Of the total amount spent for food, less than 5 per cent goes toward the purchase of fresh, dried and canned fruits. The total expenditure for fruit is 350 million dollars per year, while over one billion dollars, or 3 million dollars per day, are spent for sugar and confectionery. From statistics published by the United States Department of Agriculture, it is apparent that the average family of five now consumes about 2,500 pounds of vegetables and fruit in a year. Vegetables, which as a rule are badly prepared, make up 65 per cent of this amount, and fruits in various forms, only 35 per cent. We are actually consuming, therefore, about 175 pounds of fruit (fresh, dried and canned) per capita in a year, or less than half a pound per day. The daily amount of fresh fruit consumed amounts, on the average, to only 5 or 6 ounces per individual.

Reduced to dollars and cents, according to prices received by the producer, the daily per capita consumption of fruit in the United States is less than 1 cent; of vegetables, about 1½ cents; of refined sugar, candy and preparations artificially sweetened, about 4 cents; of cereal products, mostly demineralized, about 5 cents; and of meat and dairy products, about 12 cents. (Of course, the average amount spent daily by the individual consumer is more.) If we consider the fact that some of the fruits eaten are candied (cooked in a heavy solution of sugar) or canned and that a large part of the vegetables are also canned or cooked badly, we shall realize how surprisingly little of the alkaline elements is consumed. The daily amount of fresh fruit per individual should be about 2 pounds, while the consumption of artificial sweets, white flour products and meats should, as much as possible, be decreased, or better entirely discontinued. Consequently, the consumption of fresh and dried fruit should increase at least five times. Such an increase would be of inestimable benefit to us in every way.

Nuts—Nature's Storehouse of Fat and Protein

Nuts, the fruits of trees, bushes and plants are, botanically speaking, for the most part seeds with a more or less hard, woody covering. Many groups of plants and trees contribute to our nut supply. Deciduous trees, like the almond, pecan, walnut, chestnut, beech, hazel, etc., are the principal ones in the temperate zones. Large quantities of nuts are obtained from oaks, pines and tropical palms. The latter supply us with cocoanuts, brazilnuts, butternuts, etc., in great abundance. Others, like the peanut and pistachio, are the seeds of leguminous plants and shrubs. The sub-tropical Queensland nut is the fruit of a tall evergreen, ornamental shrub or small tree. The so-called lichi nut grown extensively in China, is really a dried fruit surrounded by a fruit-like shell. It is for sale in nearly all the Chinese stores on the Pacific Coast. The chufa, earth almond, or earth chestnut, is a perennial plant that spreads extensively by its under-ground root stocks. It bears numerous small edible tubers about the size of peanuts. The chufa belongs to the vegetable family, but as its chemical composition resembles that of nuts, it may be mentioned here. Chufas grow well upon light, sandy soils and produce large crops. The tubers, or corms, of the water-chestnut are widely used in China and Japan, and are frequently imported into the United States. Until quite recently, nuts have been used by the inhabitants of the temperate zone mostly as a luxury on special occasions, and even today the consumption is very small, as compared with the amount of other food products used. According to recent statistics, in the United States only about $50,000,000 are annually spent for nuts, or less than fifty cents per capita.

As in all seeds, the mineral matter in nuts contains a large amount of phosphoric acid, potash and magnesia, while it is deficient in sodium, lime and chlorine. The digestibility of nuts is increased if they are eaten in moderate quantities, well masticated and in combination with fruits and vegetables rich in sodium, especially green-leaf vegetables. People who live largely on meat and cereals are weakening the chemical action of the bile and pancreatic juice to such a degree that they cannot digest nuts. Moreover, nuts are often used as a dessert after a heavy meal. When eaten in this way, they are quite harmful, for they require the full action of the digestive juices. Combined with fruits or vegetable salads, nuts make a complete meal in themselves, and their indigestibility in most cases should be attributed to lack of wisdom in the choice and quantity of food eaten with them.

Nut Butters Increase the Digestibility of Nuts

Investigations made at the Yale University have proved that all nuts furnish a relatively high amount of basic amino acids, and that nut proteins are of a high biological value, fully adequate to maintain life and growth, also for the elaboration of mother's milk. Professor Cajori found in his nutrition experiments, conducted at the Sheffield laboratory, that the proteins and fats of nuts were generally absorbed to a large extent, especially when the nuts were eaten in an emulsified form as that in nut butters.

Since most people have defective teeth, they cannot reduce the entire nut by mastication into such a state that no hard pieces enter the stomach. Even small particles of such concentrated food as nuts are not easily penetrated by the digestive juices and often pass undigested through the alimentary canal. Experiments have proved that the digestibility of nuts is increased as much as ten per cent when they are taken in the form of nut butters.

Nut butters are becoming more popular every year, but most of the commercial products are made from overroasted nuts. The excessive heat develops free fatty acids and besides, the nuts are often heavily salted. Such products are not wholesome; they overtax the liver and kidneys and unduly increase the acidity of the blood. Nuts that enter into the preparation of nut butters should be dried or dehydrated at a moderate temperature, in order to make the nuts crisp, and at the same time, preserve the vitamins. Nut butters made from well-prepared, unroasted nuts rival in nutritive and hygienic value the best cuts of meat as well as cheese and dairy butter.

There is a popular belief to the effect that salting nuts prevents the digestive disturbances often arising from their indiscriminate use. To those who have acquired the salt-eating habit, nothing seems palatable without the addition of this condiment; but we know that salt interferes with the digestion of nuts, or indeed of any food.

The following table gives the average composition of nuts as compared with other foods:

Kind of Food (Edible Portion)	*Water*	*Protein*	*Fat*	*Carbo-hydrates*	*Mineral Matter*
Almond	4.9	21.4	54.4	16.8	2.5
Almond Butter	2.2	21.7	61.5	11.6	3.0
Brazil nut	4.7	17.4	65.0	9.6	3.3
Butter nut	4.5	27.9	61.2	3.4	3.0
Cashew nuts (average)	5.0	18.0	57.4	6.0	2.6
Chestnut, fresh	43.4	6.4	6.0	42.8	1.4
Chestnut, dry	6.1	10.7	7.8	73.0	2.4
Chufa	2.2	3.5	31.6	60.7	2.0
Cocoanut	13.0	6.6	56.2	22.6	1.6
Cocoanut, desiccated	3.5	6.3	57.4	31.5	1.3
Filbert	3.4	16.5	64.0	11.7	2.4
Hickory nut	3.7	15.4	67.4	11.4	2.1
Peanut	7.4	29.8	43.5	17.1	2.2
Peanut Butter	2.1	29.3	46.5	17.1	5.0
Pecan	3.4	12.1	70.7	12.2	1.6
Pine nut	3.4	14.6	61.9	17.3	2.8
Pignolia	6.2	33.9	48.2	7.9	3.8
Pistachio	4.2	22.6	54.5	15.6	3.1
Walnut	3.4	18.2	60.7	16.0	1.7
Meat, round steak	65.5	19.8	13.6	—	1.1
Cheese, cheddar	27.4	27.7	36.8	4.1	4.0
Eggs, boiled	6.5	12.4	10.7	—	0.7
Cow Butter	11.0	1.0	85.0	—	3.0
Beans, dried	12.6	22.5	1.8	59.6	3.5
Raisins	14.6	2.6	3.3	76.1	3.4
Whole Wheat Bread	35.7	8.9	1.8	52.1	1.5

The large amount of mineral matter in peanut butter and cheese is due to the table salt that has been added in their preparation.

While nuts are richest in fats, they also contain an appreciable amount of protein. The pecan contains the largest amount of fat, about 70 per cent, closely followed by the hickory nut, brazil nut, filbert and pine nut, which contain over 60 per cent of fat. The pignolia imported from Spain ranks highest in the amount of protein, containing nearly 34 per cent; the peanut comes next with 29.8 per cent; the butter nut, almond, pistachio, all contain over 20 per cent protein, excelling the best cuts of meat in that respect. The almond does not contain any starch, and is, therefore, the nut best suitable for infants, especially in the form of almond milk. The dry chestnut contains only 10 per cent protein and 70 per cent starch, and is often used in the form of chestnut flour for making bread, especially in Northern Italy and Spain. Experiments with the fruit and nut diet indicate that nut protein is as easily digested as is protein derived from bread and milk.

Nuts should constitute an integral part of the menu, rather than serve as a mere supplement to an already abundant meal. From three to four ounces of nuts well masticated, or taken in the form of unroasted nut butter, supply all the nitrogenous matter the average adult requires, without the need for other protein foods, such as eggs, cheese or meat. Moreover, the protein of nuts is of greater biological value for the renewal of the body cells than is the protein coming from the muscular tissues of a dead animal with all its wastes and poisons.

Nuts can be used with great advantage in the manufacture of real fruit candies. Four ounces of nuts ground together with twelve ounces of dried fruits, such as raisins, figs and dates make an excellent fruit confection, which is infinitely better for children than are the candies containing mostly refined sugar, often artificially colored and flavored.

Vegetables

Rich in Blood and Bone-Building Elements and Vitamins

It has been shown that if at the present time fruits were more appreciated, our supply of them would be far too small to fully meet the requirements of adequate and healthy nutrition for the nation at large. We must take more recourse to vegetables to supplement our bill of fare, especially to furnish us the needful alkaline salts and vitamins. While those who have acquired more sensible habits of eating include in their daily menu a liberal amount of salad vegetables, the mass of the American people do not as yet appreciate the great dietetic and hygienic value of the tender green leaves and stems of many plants. Only 7 per cent of the total expenditure for foods goes to the purchase of vegetables of all kinds, including canned products. But even from the comparatively small amount consumed, there is very seldom any benefit derived. The average housewife or cook boils the vegetables in too much water, and then drains them, not realizing that the larger part of the proteins, vitamins and organic salts is dissolved in the water, thereby retaining the cellulose and little else that is of real value for healthy nutrition. Then in order to replenish the loss of these most essential ingredients, table salt and spices are added to tickle the palate. Thus many tons of valuable body-building elements find their way into the sewers every year, while the drug stores do an enormous business to supply patent medicines to stimulate the jaded nervous system of a gullible public, whose impaired health is chiefly due to malnutrition.

Proper Fertilization of Vegetables Essential

Another point should be emphasized again. The nutritive and hygienic value of vegetables depends largely on the chemical composition of the soil and the kind of fertilizers that have been applied. In buying vegetables we seldom know where and in what kind of soil they have been grown. As we have explained in a previous chapter, only soil rich in the essential mineral elements can produce sound and wholesome vegetables, while manures and commercial fertilizers supply an excess of nitrogen and phosphoric acid, causing a rank and rapid growth, which misleads the inexperienced consumers. Large-sized products generally suffer from a surplus of ammonia and from a lack of alkaline bases. They have no keeping qualities and easily fall prey to disease and to insects. No sound human or animal tissues can be built from such poor vegetation, and many so-called infectious diseases have their origin in impoverished soil. Vegetables and fruits grown under proper soil conditions are delicious in flavor, very sweet, firm of flesh, deeply colored, not watery, and of course, more nutritious and wholesome. Many families could be easily supplied with good vegetables and small fruits from their own well fertilized gardens.

Proper fertilization permits closer planting and, therefore, better utilization of space. Besides, there is a certain satisfaction to be derived from raising your own well-flavored vegetables and berries that more than compensates for the labor involved.

The leaves and tender stems of vegetables, containing the largest percentage of alkaline bases, should make up a substantial part of our dietary, especially if the latter includes cereals, legumes, eggs, fish or meat. The green vegetables contain only a small percentage of solid nourishment, but they furnish a good supply of soda, lime and iron, three of the most essential alkaline elements.

The leaves, consisting of a frame work of fibrous tissue upon which the protoplasmic cells are spread out, principally serve for the respiration and nutrition of the plant, by exposing the chlorophyll-bearing cells to the air and light. The leaves also contain an appreciable amount of organic acids and vitamins. The salts enter the vegetables by their roots in the form of "ions," or electricity-charged molecules, and circulate as such through their fluids and tissues. It is here that the great importance of organic salts becomes apparent. Food in its natural condition is not merely oxidized to supply heat, but it must also furnish organic electricity in the form of negatively and positively charged ions. Perfect digestion, assimilation and elimination depend upon the presence of these electrolytes, or electrically charged ions. A constant osmotic pressure between the cells is maintained by the organic salts, which as has been repeatedly shown, play a most important part in the life processes of the body.

Fresh vegetable juices made by finely grinding the vegetables in a food chopper and pressing the pulp through a cheese cloth,* have great therapeutic value and may often be used in infant feeding. Owing to their high content of alkaline salts and mild organic acids, fresh vegetable juices are one of nature's best remedies for acidosis, which is undermining the health of many people.

Classification of Vegetables

Vegetables may be divided into five classes of which the best known are:

CLASS I. *Fruit-Bearing Vegetables*

The chayote, cucumber, eggplant, melons, okra, peppers, pumpkins, squashes and tomatoes.

CLASS II. *Green Vegetables*

Artichokes, beet-tops, brussels sprouts, cabbage, cauliflower, celery, chard, dandelion leaves, endive, ice plant, kale, lettuce, mustard leaves, New Zealand spinach, parsley, rhubarb, sorrel, spinach, watercress.

CLASS III. *Succulent Roots and Bulbs*

Asparagus, beets, carrots, celery root, chives, garlic, horseradish, kohlrabi, leek, onions, parsnips, radishes, rutabagas, salsify, turnips.

CLASS IV. *Starch-Bearing Roots and Tubers*

Arrowroot, cassava, dasheen, Jerusalem artichoke, potato, sweet potato, taro, yam, yautia.

CLASS V. *Mushrooms, Fungi, Lichens, Algae (Seaweeds)*

Of the *fruit-bearing vegetables,* cucumbers, tomatoes and the different kinds of melons are the most popular. They are best taken in their natural state, when they can exert their most beneficial influence upon the system. They contain from 90 to 95 per cent water, and while their caloric value is low, they are rich in potash, lime, magnesia and iron. To get the full benefit of these valuable alkaline elements, they should be eaten without the addition of table salt or any other condiment. The acid of the tomato, about 0.5 per cent, is mostly malic, combined with a small amount of citric and a trace of oxalic acid. The tomato, like other acid vegetables and fruits is potentially alkaline, for these

**Electrically-driven and modernly hand-operated vegetable juice extractors obviate the need for the laborious antiquated process indicated. A knowledge of the great virtues of raw vegetable juices as protective foods may be regarded as a distinctly progressive contribution to rational dietetics, answering a genuine need and filling a hitherto deeply sensed void. A large part of the nutritive value of fresh vegetables is lost by irrational preparation, particularly by overcooking. The tender leaves and stems of raw vegetables contain the largest percentage of alkaline bases, and hence they are not only essential as garnishes, but should be a substantial feature of our dietary. The majority of people, moreover, owing to defective teeth and haste in eating are hinderd in their efforts to masticate thoroughly many raw foods. and their digestive juices are not powerful enough to extract adequate nourishment therefrom.

LILLIAN R. CARQUE

acids, after being oxidized in the body, leave behind an alkaline salt. It is, therefore, a great mistake to exclude the tomato from the diet of people suffering from gout and rheumatism merely because of the trace of oxalic acid it contains. The amount is too small to have any effect upon the system. Besides, this acid always occurs in the vegetable world in combination with alkaline bases. Tomatoes, as well as cucumbers, with the addition of a few slices of green peppers, are highly beneficial in increasing the alkalinity of the blood and in removing the toxins, especially uric acid, from the system.

The *green-leaf vegetables,* which are highest in the percentage of alkaline salts, and, therefore, a most valuable addition to our diet, can nearly all be used uncooked, especially in the form of combination salads. Such vegetables as cabbage, celery, lettuce, parsley, watercress can now be procured in the larger markets nearly all the year round. Dandelion, endive, chickory, mustard greens and rhubarb can be had in the early spring and summer.

Succulent roots and bulbs contain from 75 to 90 per cent water, from 1 to 6 per cent protein and from 10 to 15 per cent carbohydrates, mostly in the form of starch and cellulose. Although they are not as rich in the alkaline elements as are the green vegetables, they contain a sufficient amount to make them valuable additions to our dietary, if properly prepared. Carrots, beets, small radishes, rutabagas and turnips contain appreciable amounts of potash, soda, lime and iron; kohlrabis, leeks and onions are particularly rich in lime, magnesia, iron and sulphur.

Asparagus is valued for its young and tender shoots, which are rich in alkaline salts and vitamins. The strong odor of the urine, after eating asparagus, is caused by a volatile oily sulphur compound. Asparagus tips may be used uncooked in combination salads.

Among the *starch-bearing tubers* the potato takes the leading place. It is a comparatively new but most valuable addition to the human bill of fare. The average composition of the potato is as follows: water 76 per cent, protein 2 per cent, starch and cellulose 21 per cent, mineral matter 1 per cent. Phosphate of potash, magnesia and chlorine constitute the larger portion of the organic salts.

The sweet potato is a true root, not a tuber. It is chiefly a produce of sub-tropical countries and an important food crop in the Gulf states, California, West India and the Philippines. It differs from the Irish potato in that its carbohydrates include considerable quantities of cane sugar and invert sugar, or glucose, which increase during storage.

Edible fungi may be divided into mushrooms, morels and truffles. The general composition of the various fungi shows that they have not a high nutritive value. The average amount of protein they contain is 3.5 per cent. The mineral matter consists mostly of phosphoric acid and potash. Truffles contain an appreciable amount of soda. They may be occasionally eaten for their flavor.

Algae include several varieties of seaweed, used as food for men and animals. The most important of these plants is *Irish moss* or *carrageen,* which is very abundant on rocky shores, especially those of Ireland. In some countries like China, Japan and the Hawaiian Islands, different kinds of seaweed are used quite extensively for food. The principal edible algae are the che choy and limu. They are rich in protein and mineral matter, especially sodium, chlorine and iodine. Another sea weed, known as *dulse* (*Rhodymenia palmata*), is found on the coast of the North Atlantic Ocean, while *kelp* (*macrocystis pyrifera*) is growing near the shores of the Pacific Ocean.

Agar-agar, known also under the name of Japanese gelatin, or sea grass, consists chiefly of a carbohydrate called "gelose," which is only soluble in hot water. Dried agar-agar in granular form is recommended for the relief of constipation because of its mechanical action on the bowels, through the expansion of the cellulose.

Cereals—Deficient in Sodium and Calcium

Cereals even in their natural state do not contain enough of the alkaline bases to prevent an increase of acidity in the blood. While they have an appreciable amount of magnesia, they are deficient in lime, soda, chlorine and often in iron and fluorine and, therefore, they do not supply enough of the elements for building sound and healthy teeth and bones. Wherever cereals are used as staple foods, they should be supplemented by a liberal amount of green-leaf vegetables to supply the necessary alkaline elements, especially sodium, calcium and iron.

The chief cereals of the world in the order of their importance are: rice, corn, wheat, oats, barley, rye, in addition to comparatively small quantities of buckwheat, millet and sorghum. The average per capita consumption of cereals by the American people is about 350 pounds, or about one pound per day for each man, woman and child. Cereals are consumed so largely because of their cheapness and the comparative ease with which they can be harvested, shipped and stored, and also because of the ever-increasing supply of so-called ready made and widely advertised breakfast foods. Incidentally it may be mentioned that about 4,800 million bushels, or 80 per cent of all cereals, are used for stock feed, serving as animal sustenance for the elaboration of meat and milk.

The chemical composition of the different cereals in their dry state is similar in water content which on an average is about 13 per cent; and also in carbohydrates (principally starch and cellulose), which range from 55 per cent in buckwheat to 71 per cent in rye. The greatest relative differences are shown in the amount of protein which is again lowest in rice, about 7 per cent and highest in some of the northern wheat, frequently as much as 17 per cent. The mineral matter varies from less than 1 per cent in rice to over 3 per cent in oats. It is a well-known fact that modern milling processes remove from 50 to 75 per cent of the organic salts, while poisonous gases are often employed in order to produce snow-white flours. Considering the enormous consumption of cereals and cereal products, these wasteful methods are most tragic in their ultimate effect upon the health and vitality of people whose diet consists largely of milling products, such as white flour, bolted corn meal, peeled and polished rice, etc. A number of children's diseases, including adenoids, swollen tonsils, caries, rickets, and in later years neuritis, pellagra and beri-beri, are aggravated by the continuous consumption of acid-forming demineralized foods.

Legumes—The Vegetable Protein Foods

Legumes include one-celled, two-valved seed pods, containing one or more seeds, such as the bean, pea and lentil. The peanut, pistachio and carob, already mentioned, also belong to the legume family. Legumes in their dry state have a very high percentage of protein ranging from 18 to 35 per cent, and even more in the case of the soy bean, which also contains from 16 to 18 per cent of fat. The composition of the mineral matter resembles that of cereals, showing a large amount of phosphate and magnesia, but it is deficient in soda, lime and iron. Only the lentil has an appreciable amount of iron. On account of their high content of proteins and carbohydrates and lack of alkaline elements, legumes are decidedly acid-forming—in fact, in the ripened seeds are stored small amounts of purin bodies. If used moderately and with discrimination, preferably with vegetable salads, legumes are a valuable and economical source of protein. The proper preparation of legumes is of great importance in order to insure their digestion and assimilation. They should be cooked in soft, distilled or rain water and preferably in a pressure cooker, which greatly reduces the time necessary to make them palatable and digestible. If the water which is used for cooking is hard, due to the presence of carbonate of lime, one teaspoonful of baking soda per gallon may be added, and then boiled and cooled before using, in order that the lime may be precipitated. If legumes are eaten too often and to excess and not in right combinations, they produce flatulency and acidity of the blood. Outdoor workers can digest legumes better than can sedentary workers, who should eat them not oftener than twice a week.

Milk, Essential for the Infant Only

Milk has been declared to be one of the essential foods to maintain health and vitality. One writer says: "Through the ages milk has been the great builder of sturdy races," while another claims that we are best nourished by including one quart of milk in our daily menu. Such assertions as these are altogether at variance with the teachings of history and physiology. There is found perhaps a greater variation in quality and chemical composition of milk than that in any other food. Nature only supplies milk for the nourishment or newborn mammals and the supply is automatically cut off after the period of lactation, which varies from one month to about one year. We cannot, therefore, say that milk is an indispensable food for the healthy growth and nutrition of the young after weaning. The rapid gain in weight during the so-called milk cure is generally impermanent. Such weight is soon lost, after one returns to one's normal diet.

Cow's milk, produced under ideal conditions, is preferable to the many artificial and demineralized foods of commerce, if it is used judiciously and supplemented by green-leaf vegetables and fruits to supply organic iron. We are not justified, however, in recommending its indiscriminate use. For milk and milk products are far from being absolute necessities for the maintenance of the health and vigor of the race. The milking of animals is an unnatural process. It lowers their vitality and often makes them victims of disease, while it impairs the quality of the milk.

Milk and dairy products are by no means staple foods with all people. The use of milk is comparatively recent in origin in the history of the human race, and even today there are people like the Japanese, who hardly take any milk.

The infant is absolutely dependent for its normal development on mother's milk, but the nursing period is comparatively short with all species of mammals, and the transition period to the food assigned to them by nature, according to their anatomical structure, is very rapid. It is evident that the nourishment a mother can supply to her newborn must be in the form of a liquid taken out of her own blood. By means of the arteries and capillaries, the blood reaches all parts of the mammary glands that secrete the wonderful fluid, which under normal conditions contains every element necessary for the proper nourishment and growth of the newborn child.

Milk, however, is not chemically akin to blood. The composition of blood is entirely different, especially in its proportion of organic salts. The sugar contained in the milk is lactose and the sugar of the blood is glucose, so that a chemical change must take place in the mammary glands.

Under normal conditions the mammary glands are active only until the teeth of the young have grown sufficiently to enable them to take care of solid food. At this period, the human body is perfectly capable of converting the natural grains, vegetables, fruits and nuts, if properly prepared, into life-giving fluids in the form of blood and lymph, which supply the system of the child with every principle required for its growth and development.

Difference in the Chemical Composition of Milk

Very little attention is generally paid to the difference in the chemical composition of milk derived from various kinds of mammals and also to the great variations existing in the composition of milk of the same animals, living under different conditions, or at different times of the year. Vitamins are not found in milk in constant quantities, and they may be almost completely lacking if the rations of the animal contain too small an amount of them. In seasons when green fodder is scarce, cows produce milk which is deficient in vitamins and alkaline salts, as compared with the milk produced when the animals are on pasture. Children's diseases, which occur most frequently in the early spring months, are most likely caused by milk produced from cows which have been poorly fed during the winter months.

Diet During Pregnancy and Lactation

Likewise mother's milk differs in organic salts and vitamins, according to the kind of food the mother eats. At times this milk may become distinctly injurious, if hygienic laws are constantly violated by the mother, or when she is subjected to strong emotions, such as fear, anger or worry. Plenty of milk and eggs are recommended to the nursing mother in order to increase the secretion of milk, but the drinking of milk does not produce milk, any more than the drinking of blood makes more blood. A diet too rich in proteins is injurious to both mother and child. Green-leaf vegetables and fresh fruits containing an abundance of alkaline salts, especially sodium, calcium, iron and vitamins, are far more essential for the production of good, nourishing milk. Mother's milk is readily affected by the use of alcoholic beverages, strong coffee, tea, narcotics and drugs, all of which should be avoided during pregnancy. It is a great mistake for the pregnant mother to think she must eat enough for two. In fact, overeating is the cause of many miscarriages and also of insufficient lactation.

Faulty diet of the nursing mother and consequently inadequate feeding of infants is one of the greatest sources of human suffering and inefficiency in later life, because it means lessened vitality and power of resistance. Until recently it was taken for granted that whatever milk was formed by the mammary glands of the nursing mother was good for the baby. We know that the quality of mother's milk is absolutely dependent on the food she eats and the state of her emotions, not only during the nursing period, but also during pregnancy. There is nothing more essential for the prospective mother than is the study of rational dietetics as outlined in this little volume.

Substitutes for Mother's Milk

Various formulae intended to replace human milk by modified cow's milk have been extolled, but they can never imitate the highly organized compounds which nature has evolved in her own laboratory and which are best adapted to the healthy growth of the new-born infant. So-called modified cow's milk may appear to be a good imitation of human milk, but the fact remains that there always is a discrepancy in organic constituents, especially in regard to the quality of the casein and proportion of organic salts. Although many infants may effect an immediate gain in weight and fatten the infant, these seeming changes for the better are usually produced at the expense of its vitality.

Overfeeding the Cause of Tonsilitis

Overfeeding and the indiscriminate use of substitutes for mother's milk are the most frequent mistakes in the rearing of infants, and a large number of so-called infantile diseases are due to these causes. Many of the older children are overfed with cow's milk, which is generally pasteurized and taken together with all kinds of devitalized starchy foods and often meat. Nearly all cases of tonsilitis are the result of an irrational diet, which overloads the system with waste poisons. The lymphatic glands in the neck, which have to neutralize the toxic acids, soon break down from overwork and become swollen, and then the bloodstream empties its toxins into the membranes of the ear and nose, causing dullness of mind and pathological conditions in the body. The removal of tonsils and adenoids has become quite fashionable, but these very operations do not remove the cause of the evil, namely toxemia or acidosis, due to wrong feeding. While under present conditions milk as food for children should not be condemned altogether, it should always be taken with discrimination and by itself, and not hastily consumed with incompatible mixtures of other foods. The more extensive use of fruits and nuts should gradually reduce the great consumption of milk and dairy products.

Dairy Products

Butter is preferable to oleomargarines, as it contains some vitamins and organic salts derived from the milk, which are lacking in most of the hydrogenated vegetable oils.* The analysis of butter shows 11 per cent water, 1 per cent protein, 85 per cent fat and 3 per cent mineral matter. Most of the butter is heavily salted in order to preserve it. Fresh sweet butter is much more wholesome.

Cheese is another popular dairy product. It is made from curdled milk, more or less skimmed by the action of the rennet, which turns the casein into a solid state in which a large part of the fat and organic salts are retained. In the process of ripening cheese, a portion of the casein is peptonized, while at the same time some odoriferous substances are formed, which give to each variety of cheese its peculiar taste and flavor. These vary according to the nature of the bacteria, which are active in the ripening of the curd. All cheeses are concentrated foods, rich in casein, fat and phosphate of lime; on the average they contain from 25 to 35 per cent of casein and albumen and from 15 to 30 per cent of fat. Nearly all cheeses are heavily salted. Fresh cottage cheese, made from whole milk, unsalted, is the most wholesome cheese. It contains about 20 per cent of casein, 1 per cent lactose and lactic acid, 4.3 per cent fat, and 1.8 per cent mineral matter, rich in phosphate of lime. It rivals in nutritive value the best cuts of meat and is free from animal waste matter.

Eggs

Eggs, despite the enormous consumption of dairy products in modern times, were a late addition to the human bill of fare, although primitive man may have occasionally eaten birds' eggs. Like the seeds of cereals and legumes, each fertile egg contains a germ or embryo bird until it has reached a stage in its development that life outside the confinement of the cell becomes possible.

**Oleomargarines are now fortified with added vitamins.

LILLIAN R. CARQUE

The embryo is in close relation with the yolk, the white being used later. The yolk and white of the egg must naturally differ in chemical composition, according to the purpose served. The whole egg contains about 74 per cent water, 12.5 per cent protein, 12 per cent fat and 1.1 per cent mineral matter. The yolk has about 51 per cent water, 16 per cent protein, 32 per cent fat, and 1.1 per cent mineral matter. The yolk is richer in iron than is the white, as it has to supply the blood for the chick. Eggs have an excess of nitrogen, fat and phosphoric acid, and are consequently acid-forming. For this reason eggs should be used in moderation, no more than two or three times a week, and then always combined with vegetables or fruits which are strongly alkaline, preferably salads made from green-leaf vegetables. In boiling or frying the eggs the albumen begins to coagulate at a temperature of 160° F. and becomes white, opaque and insoluble in water. The nutritive value of eggs is generally overestimated; they are three parts water against one part solid matter; 32 eggs are required to make one pound of water-free food material.

Meat—The Least Essential and Most Expensive Food

Few people realize that the slaughtering of animals for food is one of the largest industries in the United States, and that the value of its annual products amounts to over two billion dollars. This, of course, is the total received by the meat packers; the actual amount paid by consumers is perhaps four times as much. There are over 1,600 large slaughter houses, besides many more smaller establishments throughout the country. Over 120 million four-footed animals are killed every year; and this number does not include animals slaughtered by butchers in small towns or on farms, or killed by hunters. The meat-packing industry began with a small pork-packing establishment in Cincinnati about fifty years ago, and only since then has developed to its present magnitude. The per capita consumption of meat in the United States was 145 pounds in 1921, having declined about 20 pounds per capita since 1900. It is steadily declining since 1924. Only three countries exceed the United States in meat consumption, namely Australia, New Zealand and Argentine, with over 200 pounds per capita consumption in each country. In Europe the average annual per capita consumption is about 70 pounds. It is highest in Great Britain and lowest in Italy. The per capita consumption in large cities is much higher than that in the country. Japan has the lowest per capita of consumption of all countries: 1.5 pounds of meat and 25 pounds of fish.

Meat-eating originated comparatively late in the history of man's evolution, and it appears that this deviation from his natural diet was by no means voluntary, but caused by extreme want. The man who was first driven by fierce hunger to kill an animal and eat the meat certainly did not find it a palatable meal, and it probably made him feel miserable afterwards as a boy after he has smoked his first cigar. Under the pressure of famine, caused by inundations of large stretches of land and mighty geological cataclysms during the glacial era, man was forced to take recourse to flesh foods.

Mankind's cradle was undoubtedly located in the tropics, where vegetation is most productive, and where an abundant supply of fruits, nuts and succulent plants could be procured throughout the year. Geological research has succeeded in tracing man's ancestry back to the middle and even to the early part of the tertiary period.

It is likely that the use of flesh foods originated during long periods of scarcity, when no other foods were available, and that it was during this time that man, after he had invented the first crude stone weapons, first became a hunter. While the consumption of flesh foods for many thousands of years may indeed have given to man certain carnivorous characteristics, yet his *anatomical structure and physiological functions remain unchanged.* This conclusively proves that nature designed him to be a fruit eater. Eventually he will return to a diet consisting largely of fruits, much improved in nutritive and hygienic value by special cross-pollenation and intelligent cultivation of the soil.

Meat Protein Subject to a Rapid Putrefaction

Those who assert that meat is a superior food should note the marked physiological differences between the products of the vegetable kingdom and those of flesh foods. In the vegetable organism the constructive forces are at work combining inorganic materials into complex organic compounds and storing them in its own tissues. In the animal organism the constructive and destructive forces are simultaneously active. In the blood and tissues of the dead animal we find numerous substances in the process of disintegration. These waste products are poisonous and must be quickly eliminated from the system.

Extended research has established the fact that meat protein is twice as putrescible as is vegetable protein. The proteins of fresh meat may be more easily digested, but for the final reconstructive and eliminative processes of our body cells they are inferior to the proteins in fresh fruits, green-leaf vegetables and nuts. It has further been proved that, even after having been acted upon by the digestive juices, proteins of vegetable origin are much less putrescible than are those of meat. The rapid putrefaction of the latter is undoubtedly due to its unstable chemical composition, as it is not combined with sufficient alkaline elements, especially those of lime and sodium. *Of all foods meat is by far the most toxic, and death can be much hastened by the administration of it to a sick creature.*

The people of the Occident still cling tenaciously to the belief that meat is their best food because they have been taught false dietary standards. Our medical textbooks still contain many erroneous ideas about foods and nutrition. Of course, there are those who are influenced by habit, fashion, or unfavorable environment to make meat the largest part of their diet, but we have no scientific proof that such people excel in mental and physical development merely because they happen to consume large quantities of flesh foods. The people inhabiting the Arctic zones, who subsist almost exclusively on animal food products, are under-sized and short-lived. They could not exist at all, if they did not take certain precautions to counteract, at least to some extent, the effects of protein poisoning. Many green herbs and salmon-berries are eagerly consumed during the short summer season. A seaweed common in the north is eaten in large quantities. The Eskimo eats his meat raw without the addition of salt and condiments; he uses the animal's blood and internal organs which contain some vitamins and mineral elements lacking in the muscular tissues; he also partakes of a large amount of fat.

There is no ingredient in meat which we cannot procure in better quality from the thousand and more products of the vegetable kingdom. Meat, at its very best, is an expensive food material, insufficient for the formation of healthy blood and tissues. Lean meat, on the average, contains about 72 per cent water, 20 per cent protein, 5 per cent fat, 2 per cent extractive matters and 1 per cent mineral matter. The protein is made up of a number of amino acids, but not sufficient for proper growth. Lean meat is deficient in vitamins "A" and "B", and contains only a small amount of vitamin "C". It has, therefore, little anti-scorbutic value. Tinned and pickled meats are practically valueless in this respect. The extractive matters contain most of the waste poisons, which give meat its stimulating effect, generally mistaken for strength-giving properties. Meat is especially deficient in sodium, calcium and iron. What iron is found in it is due to the small amount of blood retained in the muscular tissues. This iron is inferior in biological value to the iron compounds of fruits and vegetables, built up directly by the actinic rays of the sunlight.

Wastefulness of Meat Production

Another and perhaps the most important and far-reaching argument in favor of a meatless diet, is that man can derive his nourishment from a much smaller area when living on the products of the soil, for he then receives them immediately from nature, instead of feeding them first to cattle and then living on their flesh. As the population of the earth steadily increases, man will have to content himself with a proportionately smaller area on which to raise his food supply. The land now serving for hunting grounds and cattle raising could be much more economically utilized for the cultivation of fruits, nuts and vegetables. It has been estimated that a given tract of well-cultivated land can sustain at least twenty times more people by its crops than can be nourished on the meat of cattle that feed on the vegetation growing in the same area. In the temperate zones of the American Continent and in Europe the chief object of agriculture is the cultivation of certain cereals and vegetables as food for animals intended for meat-production, instead of providing man directly with suitable and wholesome products of the soil.**

**Let us hope that the newly inaugurated system of tank or soilless gardening through the agencies of water and minerals will bring agriculture under greater scientific control, and will serve as an economic factor in small scale production.

LILLIAN R. CARQUE

Investigations have shown that an ox of average size daily eats during the winter from 45 to 50 pounds of different kinds of fodder, including about 20 pounds corn-silage. On such a ration about 1½ pounds of edible muscular tissues are produced per day. In other words we have to give an ox 30 pounds of food material in order to produce 1 pound of meat. We may assume that the land necessary for feeding one ox could, under intensive cultivation, produce enough fruits, nuts and vegetables to support ten people.

The wastefulness of meat production from the standpoint of national resources is well stated by Professor Armsby, a leading authority on animal nutrition:

> "It may be roughly estimated that about 24 per cent of the energy of grain is recovered for consumption in pork, about 18 per cent in milk, and only about 3.5 per cent in beef and mutton. In other words, the farmer who feeds bread grains to his stock is burning up 75 to 97 per cent of them in order to produce for us a small residue of roast pig or beefsteak; and so diminishes the total stock of human food."

Professor O. E. Baker of the United States Department of Agriculture, in a notable paper read before the Association of American Geographers in April, 1922, said:

> "Fully three-fifths of the crop acreage in the United States is used to produce feed for farm animals; and in addition, our live stock consume the products of about 75 million acres of improved pasture; probably of 150 million acres of unimproved grassland and pasture in farms, and about 200 million acres of woodland pasture in farms and in our national forests, besides that of perhaps 500 million acres of arid or semi-arid open range land in the West. It seems safe to say that the live stock consume two-thirds of the product of improved land and practically all the product of the unimproved pasture or fully 80 per cent of the total food and feed produced by tame and wild vegetation in the United States."

Our Wrong System of Agriculture

Public health cannot profit very much from a system of feeding which is based upon our present system of agriculture. The principal and often excessive consumption of meat and cereals and the consequent craving for stimulants and narcotics, is the chief cause of an almost universal toxemic condition and a social unrest of the people, frequently intensified by over production and unemployment in the industrial fields. Today we are devoting over 200 million acres to the cultivation of the different cereals. The total harvest is approximately 5 billion bushels, most of which goes to the feeding of 20 millions of animals. Only a comparatively small proportion of the developed agricultural land is devoted to the cultivation of fruits, nuts and vegetables. Cereals and meat are not the best foods for man. In fact, he could live much better by reducing their consumption to a minimum and by eating more fruits, nuts and vegetables instead, supplemented occasionally by small amounts of dairy products, such as buttermilk, clabbermilk or cottage cheese.

The Importance of Fruit Culture

In the progress of civilization, fruit and nut trees will always be a necessary and important element, not only to provide wholesome and ample nourishment, but also to enhance man's love for the beauties of nature. Mineral substances can be drawn from greater depths by fruit and nut trees than those which can be extracted by cereals, as the strong roots of trees are capable of reaching the deeper, richer strata of the soil, permitting therefore a more intensive cultivation of a given area of land.

Agriculture and horticulture are the most natural and wholesome occupations of man, the foundation of all other occupations. In a nation wishing to achieve a healthy organism, about seventy-five per cent of the population should occupy themselves largely with progressive and wholesome agricultural and horticultural activities, the free arts and cultural pursuits, and twenty-five per cent with trades and commerce.

For health and delight, the garden and the orchard are the universal and supreme ideal of man. The love of country and orchard is the one abiding memory of an almost forgotten paradise. How beautiful is the sight of an orchard, with its blooming trees sending their roots deep down into the soil, drinking in the heavenly light with its millions of blossoms bringing forth the luscious fruits in which the hidden treasures of the earth and the life-giving forces of the sun are so wonderfully combined!

Man will cling to the land; he will see that it is the earth which nourishes him best, and, like the giant Antaeus, he will ever have need to touch it, to feel it beneath his feet, in order to renew his strength. The time will surely come when science and co-operation of mankind will have cultivated the earth to such a degree that it will bring ample nourishment, happiness, and contentment for all. Then the shadows of disease, famine, murder, and war will disappear from our planet like the mists of night before the radiant rays of the rising sun.

CHAPTER XV

ALKALINE AND ACID-FORMING FOODS

The American people annually spend over twenty billion dollars for food materials. Of this sum, the foods which supply the acid-binding or alkaline elements in sufficient quantity make up only 12 per cent of the total expenditure. But attention should be called to the fact that vegetables in America are generally prepared in such a manner that they lose a large proportion of their essential organic salts. Large quantities of canned fruits are used, in which syrup made from refined sugar is added. Cow's milk may be considered as a natural food, but becomes acid-forming when boiled or sterilized. Meat, eggs, cheese, cereals, sugar, all acid-forming foods, make up over 75 per cent of our food supply, with the result that most people suffer from acidosis, or acidity of the blood. Our diet should be just the reverse. We should consume five times more of fruits and vegetables, preferably in their natural state, and only a small amount of the more concentrated foods like cereals, nuts and dairy products, while refined sugar and white flour should be discarded altogether.

The *base-forming or alkaline foods are*: fresh fruits and unsulphured dried fruits, green-leaf and root vegetables, potatoes, if baked, and milk if taken in its natural state, as it comes from the animal; the casein of pasteurized, boiled and sterilized milk becomes coagulated according to the degree of heat applied. Buttermilk has an alkaline reaction.

In the anti-toxic diet the proportion of the alkaline to that of the acid-forming elements should be about four to one. Sodium is one of the most powerful solvents, especially for the removal of carbonic acid, but it is one of the alkaline elements which are usually furnished in an insufficient quantity. If our diet is strongly alkaline, we can live well on a surprisingly low amount of protein. This is a very important fact when we consider that most of the bodily ailments which deplete our vital force come from auto-intoxication, the self-poisoning resulting from eating too much protein and a deficiency of organic salts in our foods.

As indicated, the best way to properly arrange our diet is to divide the available foods into base-forming and acid-forming, and to use a larger proportion of the former with as little artificial preparation as possible.

The *acid-forming foods are*: flesh foods and fish of all kinds, eggs and cheese, cereals and cereal products, legumes, nuts, especially roasted nuts, heavily sulphured fruits and fruits preserved in syrup, refined sugar, candy, confectionery, chocolate, cocoa, butter, margarine, lard and hydrogenated oils, coffee, tea, artificially sweetened and colored soft drinks and alcoholic beverages of all kinds.

Mistakes in Classification of Foods

Quite a few writers on dietetics make the mistake of classifying such foods as beans, lima beans, almonds, etc., as base-forming because they have a preponderance of alkaline minerals which leave behind a basic ash residue in the final end processes of metabolism. We must remember, however, that the alkalinity or acidity of foods is also determined by the amount of protein, starch, sugar and of fats they contain, all of which leave an acid reaction.

Vegetables, especially the green leaves, all kinds of fruit and raw milk, are the only really alkaline foods, because they are comparatively low in protein, carbohydrates and fat, while they are rich in alkaline elements. The term, *acidosis,* is really a misnomer. It merely indicates that the body's alkalinity is rather below normal, for if the body became actually acid even in a small degree, death would result.

There are certain fruits which contain a very small amount of benzoic acid, for example, cranberries, plums and prunes. This, however, does not diminish their alkaline value as foods. The trace of benzoic acid contained in these fruits is combined in the kidneys with glycocoll or glycin (an amino acid) and is eliminated in the urine as hippuric acid. Foods preserved with artificially synthetized benzoic acid should, of course, be avoided, since all anti-ferments interfere with digestion and assimilation.

Tomatoes have also been erroneously classified as an acid-forming food, on account of their oxalic acid content. The amount of this acid usually contained in tomatoes does not exceed 0.5 parts in 10,000, while citric and malic acids amount to about 0.5 per cent. Nevertheless, tomatoes are strongly alkaline, as they are rich in potassium, sodium, calcium and iron. Oxalic acid is contained in varying amounts in many fruits and vegetables (from 0.01 to 3 parts in 1,000 parts of fresh substance). If the blood has an alkaline reaction, oxalic acid is readily neutralized and eliminated, but in case of acidosis a part of the oxalic acid may pass into the kidneys unchanged, giving rise to the formation of calcium oxalate stones in the kidneys and bladder. The primary cause of this pathological condition is the excessive consumption of meat, cheese, cereals, legumes, etc., which are all highly acid-forming.

Cocoa and black tea (in their dry state) show the highest amount of oxalic acid and over-indulgence in the decoctions made therefrom, combined with an acid-forming diet, greatly favor the formation of kidney and bladder stones (calculi).

The natural way to dissolve and excrete these mineral deposits from the body is to reduce the amount of acid-forming foods to a minimum, and to live mostly on fresh fruits and green-leaf vegetables in the form of combination salads.

Many popular drugs lessen the alkalinity of the blood. The freely-used aspirin is one of the commonest offenders. Aspirin is a pain killer and when given for headaches, for example, temporarily checks the pain. But as soon as the effect of the drug wears off, the headache may be even worse, due to the added acidosis produced by the drug.

All artificial and highly concentrated foods often containing poisonous preservatives, prevent the formation of healthy blood and normal digestive juices, and therefore, interfere with the normal nutritional processes of the body.

Raw and Cooked Food

Although the advocates of raw food as an exclusive diet have many arguments in their favor, yet, under the present conditions of living, not everybody can suddenly change from a diet of mostly cooked foods to one of raw food only. Cooking of food probably originated during the last glacial period, or at least 30,000 years ago, and has been practiced more or less since the making of fire was invented by man. However, primitive man did not deprive his food of the essential mineral elements while preparing it. The extensive manufacture of denatured foods with its fatal consequences upon the health of man is one of the characteristics of our present commercial age, especially of the last fifty years. The injurious and degenerating effects of the ever-increasing consumption of impoverished, preserved, pickled and adulterated foods, combined with an intensified craving for stimulants and narcotics, will make themselves more and more felt by the coming generations, unless people awaken to the great importance of food reform and adopt saner methods of living and thinking.

The change in our diet should be made gradually and intelligently, always considering our state of health and the conditions under which we have to live at present. By subsisting for many centuries largely on cooked foods and by depriving ourselves of the necessary out-of-door exercise, the digestive organs of civilized man have become more or less weakened, so that in many cases he cannot suddenly change to a diet of uncooked foods, especially cereals, fibrous and starchy vegetables, without much inconvenience. We must begin with discarding all denatured products and prepare our foods without robbing them of the essential organic salts.

There is no doubt that cooking, especially if prolonged, renders all food less valuable. But we should remember that the majority of persons, owing to their imperfect teeth, cannot thoroughly masticate many raw foods, and their digestive juices are not strong enough to extract adequate nourishment therefrom.

If cooking is employed at all, it should be done with modern steam-cooking utensils which enable us to quickly soften the cellulose covering the cell walls of vegetables without immersing them in water. By this method only a very small part of their nutritive value is lost, and we make them more palatable and also more accessible to the digestive juices.

CHAPTER XVI

FUNDAMENTAL FACTS ABOUT HEALTH AND DISEASE IN THE LIGHT OF MODERN BIOLOGY

What is Disease?

Throughout the organic world we find the life principle always asserting itself. Our inherent vital force is constantly trying to preserve life at all costs and only gives up the struggle when the obstructions put across its path become too tremendous and overwhelming to be overcome. We cannot emphasize the fact too strongly that what we call "disease" is really a process of purification on the part of the system—a special effort of the organism to burn up and throw off abnormal quantities of waste poisons that have their origin in our perverted dietetic and hygienic habits, resulting from false teachings and erroneous thinking. *Nature does not provide any specific remedies for specific diseases.* She inflicts penalties for every transgression of her laws. She warns us in time with her red flag signals, usually in the form of catarrh, inflammation, pain, etc. But these warnings are, as a rule, not heeded or are misunderstood, due to ignorance and the misinformation that is being daily broadcasted in our schools, magazines and newspapers. When abnormal conditions arise in our organism, the fundamental cause must be found, which in the majority of cases is within ourselves—the result of wrong living and thinking.

Mankind has not yet awakened to the fact that the body is an organic whole; that in the last analysis diseases have one common source—diminished vital force or enervation, resulting from the retention of waste poisons; that pain is but a local symptom of general disorder; and that, finally, *if any real and permanent relief is to be attained, successful treatment cannot consist in confining one's efforts exclusively to the organ or part affected, but the organism must be treated in its entirety.*

The majority of people do not know what real health and vitality mean because they never actually enjoy them. Their vitality is always below par on account of their constant violation of the laws of their being. Indispositions are regarded as a matter of course and are believed to be caused by the weather, so-called germs of disease, or other external conditions. To be sure, our present social and economic system, which is largely upheld by greed and selfishness, and which has for its highest goal the accumulation of material wealth, is also responsible to a large extent for the neglect of hygienic measures, and the resulting enervation that seems to afflict civilized mankind in an ever increasing degree.

Health and disease are not diametrically opposed to each other. Disease is not something that suddenly attacks us from without, like a thunderbolt from a clear sky, or like a carnivorous animal jumping upon its prey. Disease is simply an attempt on the part of *vis medicatrix naturae* (nature's healing power) to restore normal conditions in the organism. Every acute disease such as fever, catarrh, cold, etc., is an effort at body-cleaning, and all that nature needs is to be left alone. At least, only such measures should be adopted as will assist nature in her work of eliminating poisonous waste matter. Fasting for several days, cleansing the colon, resorting to water applications and adopting a restricted diet under the supervision of an intelligent nature cure physician will generally bring quick relief.

It should be remembered, however, that the *determination of the patient to get well and his faith in nature's healing forces will greatly help to restore health and vitality.* Any obstruction of nature's efforts by the use of poisonous drugs and serums, or by forcing food on the patient will only impede recovery. It often proves fatal by lowering his vitality and by increasing the work of the heart and the eliminative organs. Drug and serum treatment is responsible for thousands of chronic ailments and premature deaths, and yet it is sanctioned by law.

The Delusive Action of Drugs and Serums

Drugs and serums, whether of animal, vegetable or mineral origin, have only a temporary stimulating effect, in so far as they are acted upon by the inherent vital force of the body in its defense against these poisons. This defensive action of the organism is generally mistaken as a beneficial influence of the specific remedy, which in the majority of cases leads to the formation of the drug habit and to the gradual lowering of vitality and of the power of resistance.

Drug poisons always interfere with the synthetic processes of the living cell, causing disintegration and break down of the tissues faster than they can be rebuilt by the inherent vital force. By drug and serum treatment, the organism becomes so weakened, that a large part of the drugs will be retained in the tissues, laying the foundation for chronic ailments and for premature death. Hundreds of new pharmaceutical preparations are thrown upon the market every year, millions of dollars are spent for advertising them, and the credulous public pays not only the bills, but also takes in exchange impaired health and lowered vitality.**

The popular sedatives and pain killers, such as *bromides, aspirin, acetanilid, phenacetin, phenol phtalein* (mostly used in laxative pills and tablets) and many other coal tar products, endorsed by the medical profession, generally interfere with autonomic brain centers and act as permanent depressants, often with fatal results.

One of the most insiduous and widely used drugs is *quinine,* a poisonous alkaloid, extracted from the bark of the Cinchona tree, and prescribed as an

**Rational living, lofty morals and high thinking will ultimately produce in any individual a blood-stream immune to every disease. But what an arduous long-drawn-out task, involving self-discipline, introspection, as well as a certain amount of suffering along with rigid dietetic and moral self-denials!

LILLIAN R. CARQUE

antipyretic especially in cases of colds and fevers; while it may bring immediate results, it will in time severely affect the brain and nervous system. It has a paralyzing effect upon the digestive tract and reduces fever by suppressing the vital functions. Some of the characteristic symptoms of quinine poisoning are nervous irritability, extreme mental depression (melancholia), ringing in the ears and serious visual disturbances. The delusive action of quinine is characteristic of many other drugs, for which a misguided and misinformed public spends millions of dollars every year.

The tremendous growth of the drug industry in the United States is a positive proof of the inability of the majority of medical practitioners to treat their patients in a rational and efficient manner. During the last thirty years over forty thousand new remedies have been put on the market and their number is constantly increasing. *Cures,* like fashions, have come and gone. Such dubious remedies as anti-toxins, tuberculin, turtle's blood, salvarsan and a hundred others have been heralded to a suffering world as wonderful discoveries of medical science, only to be abandoned after a brief period as unsatisfactory.

The majority of people have yet to learn that lasting health can only come through a true understanding of the normal functions of the body, and through an application of simple and rational methods for maintaining them in a healthy condition. Because a few who have inherited a large amount of vitality are able, with apparent impunity, to defy the laws of nature for some time, many are disposed to sneer at rational methods of living. As a rule, however, death claims them when they have attained the age of fifty of sixty (and sometimes earlier), when man's mental powers and his general usefulness to humanity should be at their maximum.

The Germ Theory of Disease

The theory that diseases such as meningitis, diphtheria, influenza, typhoid fever and tuberculosis are directly caused by germs has arisen from a lack of understanding of the laws of biology and physiological chemistry. The germ theory of disease is erroneous in all of its aspects. The human cell is the result of millions of years of evolution and has, therefore, a much higher organization than have the so-called germs of disease, which are simply scavengers, feeding only on the devitalized or dying cells and on the waste products of our system, but never on healthy, living cells, which are impervious to the attack of bacteria.

The French chemist, Louis Pasteur, while investigating the cause of the fermentation of fruit juices and malt liquors, discovered a number of different germs, known as yeast cells, which by their rapid growth and development effected chemical changes in the liquid, the principal change being the conversion of sugar into alcohol and into carbonic acid. Pasteur, who compared the living body to a vat of fermentable liquid, conceived the idea that our organism was likewise at the mercy of various extraneous microbes. He believed the different germs to be individual entities, endowed with well-defined functions, and propounded the doctrine of specific malignant, atmospheric germs, each causing a specific malady. If we analyze these assumptions, we find that Pasteur tried to reverse the process of evolution in the organic world in predicting that the lowest form of life can successfully attack the highest form—the living human cell.

The laboratory study of fermentation is by no means original with Pasteur. It is now an established fact that Pasteur appropriated many of the ideas and discoveries which made him famous from the teachings of his contemporary, Professor Antoine Bechamp.

It was Bechamp's idea that cells or germs were no more than transitory organic units, built up by numerous still smaller entities which he called microzyma, or minute, ferment-bodies. He maintained that the processes of putrefaction are the result of the action of these microzyma, which are set free as the life of their habitat, the organic cell, comes to an end; and further, that all the micro-organisms found in the air and soil are the remains of animal and vegetable matter. Bechamp's contention is supported by the fact that bacteria abound wherever decaying organic matter is found, that micro-organisms are almost totally absent on the tops of high mountains or in the sterile sand and dry air of the large deserts. Briefly, Bechamp's theory is this: vegetable and animal cells are made up of microzyma which are set free as the former disintegrate. The microzyma of animal cells, when originating in morbid matter, form themselves into bacteria. The latter are the products of so-called disease and not the cause of it. To quote Bechamp:

> "Disease is born of us and in us and that is as it should be, because the life of man, and of every other creature, is no more delivered over to chance than the course of the stars. Life would be delivered over to chance if it depended upon primitive microbic germs created for destructive purposes."

Bechamp's views were shared by that eminent German physiologist, Rudolf Virchow, who said towards the end of his remarkable career:

> "If I could live my life over again I would devote it to proving that germs seek their natural habitat, diseased tissue. rather than being the cause of the diseased tissue."

Why Bacteriology is Misleading

Until Pasteur gave the germ theory to the profession, cause of disease was ascribed to many things: evil spirits, mists in the air, plethory, humors in the blood, miasma, etc. These beliefs still linger along with a belief in germs.

In fifty years of intensively exploiting the germ theory, there is not one disease that has been proved positively to be of germ origin and not one that can be cured according to the germ theory. Unless a germ will produce a disease every time it enters the body, it is not a cause. A cause must be constant and specific in its influence, or it is not a cause. Germs are omnipresent. This is one of the fundamental truths that Pasteur discovered; but he and his followers appear to have overlooked the fact that germs fail to have a specific influence all the time. Germs cause fermentation in fruit juices under the proper environment and temperatures, between 50 and 110 degrees Fahrenheit. Fermentation takes place when the fruit is bruised and the skin is broken; but when the covering—the skin or rind—is unbroken, some fruits dry up and are preserved; or when the skin is removed or the fruit cut in halves and dehydrated, the germs fail to set up fermentation, on account of the greatly reduced moisture content of the fruit.

The fundamental hypothesis that germs cause disease has never been proved. Hence bacteriology is not true, and that part of medical science resting on that hypothesis must be abandoned. How long it will take the cobhouse to come down is hard to say, for it rests on a solid commercial foundation.

That after more than fifty years of trying out the germ idea of disease it has not been verified, indicates that it never will be. The trial has been thorough. Every scientist and every scientific fact have been used in trying to prove the hypothesis, and every supposed victory in proof of the theory has been heralded and adopted and public opinion coerced; and then it has been abandoned for another. These discoveries have followed each other in rapid succession—rapidly enough to discourage the most hopeful.

Why all these failures? Because Pasteur was a chemist and laboratory worker. If he had been a physician and biochemist with years of practical experience at the bedside, he would, with his wonderfully analytical mind, have learned that a normal man is immune to the action of germs, and that the germ action is always secondary; that when germs invade a living organism it is a sign that the organism is enervated and its chemistry perverted. He proved that germs caused the juice of fruit in an open vat to ferment, but he did not prove that the juice as it exists in the fruit would ferment without a cause.

Fruits, vegetables, animals and man have an innate power to resist the influence of germs. When resistance is lost and the chemistry is thrown out of balance, then disorganizing bacteriological fermentation starts up at some vulnerable point. The normal man has more physical resistance than has all life below him; and in addition, he has a mental equipment that multiplies his power of resistance.

Microbes or bacteria are really the scavengers of the animal and human body, found only in decaying cells and waste matter, but never attacking healthy living cells. They cannot, from the standpoint of medical science, be regarded as the cause of diseases, for if this were the case, we should all, whether sick or well, become victims of one or more germ diseases, in spite of immunization and the most rigid quarantine. Germs are everywhere. They are indispensable to the development of the higher forms of life. If it were possible to exterminate all the microbes of this planet, organic life would come to an end.

Yet for the past sixty years the medical profession has been led astray by looking for the cause and cure of disease through bacteriology instead of through biochemistry and regenerated thoughts and motives.

Diminished alkalinity of the body fluid—blood and lymph—and tissues, including bone and nerve tissue, is the turning point, the line of demarcation between health and disease because it impairs function and structure, leading to the formation of cellular poisons along with the incidental growth and multiplication of bacteria.

Dr. Koch's Discovery Abandoned

When Pasteur propagated his theory first of all, Professor Koch of Berlin, discoverer of *tuberculin* as a cure for tuberculosis, said:

"If it is true, then there are four postulates that must be complied with. If there is a specific germ which is the cause of the specific disease, it must always be found in connection with that disease. Secondly, it ought not to be found apart from the disease. Thirdly, we ought to be able to cultivate it apart from the human body, and fourthly, when inoculated into an animal it should produce a disease synonymous with that which obtains in the human body."

Those postulates as a whole have never been complied with yet in any one single disease supposed to be originated by a germ. Therefore, there is no scientific significance in the germ theory of disease, and the whole superstructure of vaccines and serums must fall to the ground like a house of cards. Latterly the bacteriologists are altering their views. Monsieur Henri of the Pasteur Institute has declared that these germs change their shape in a most remarkable way, and that under the influence of violet rays a round germ was changed into a long bacillus, and that when a cultivation of the latter was inoculated into an animal, the effect produced was quite different from what it was when it was in its round shape. This shows there can be no such thing as a specific germ causing a specific disease.

Today, forty years from Koch's discovery, we have a startling report on February 17, 1933, by Dr. H. J. Corper, director of research in the National Jewish Hospital in Denver, speaking before a joint meeting of the Colorado Tuberculosis Association, the Denver Sanitarium Association, the El Paso County Sanitarium Association, and the Denver County Medical Society. He had the following to say:

"Much of our information regarding tuberculosis is hypothetical, and our treatment of that disease today is founded merely on theory."

In pointing out what he termed "our fundamental lack of knowledge regarding tuberculosis," Dr. Corper said his purpose was not to cast reflection upon what already has been accomplished, but to show how much there was yet to be done.

"Research has proved that the prevalent belief that tuberculosis germs are present in the blood of those suffering from the disease is unfounded," he said. "Tests show the germs are not found in the blood of even advanced cases."

"The occasional spread of the disease from one region of the body to another by way of the blood results from purely accidental and rare discharge of broken-down tuberculosis pus into a blood-vessel. The germs quickly are removed from the bloodstream by lodging in some other organ."

"Stamping Out" Disease

The attempt to "stamp out" disease will be futile as long as people violate the laws of hygiene. At the present time more persons than ever before die at an age when they ought to be functioning at their best. The mortality rate after the age of 40 has greatly increased in the last fifty years. Vital statistics show that every year 366,000 persons in this country die before the age of 30; 449,000 before the age of 40; 543,000 before the age of 50; 655,000 before the age of 60; 786,000 before the age of 70; and 919,000 before the age of 80. These mortality rates will increase as long as personal and public hygiene is neglected.

Seventy-five years ago, the great pioneer of Nature Cure in the United States, Dr. R. T. Trall, asked this pertinent question:

"Why has not success in treating diseases kept pace with the extraordinary progress of knowledge in related sciences? The answer is ready: a successful practice of the healing art must be based upon the laws of life, the economy of vitality. The only foundation, therefore, of true medical practice is correct physiological principles; and here is precisely where the whole orthodox medical system of the present day fails—utterly and totally fails. It has no physiological and biological science upon which to truly practice the healing art."

These words are equally applicable today. After half a century of medical practice, Dr. J. H. Tilden says in his "Philosophy of Health":

"In spite of the greatest perfection attained in diagnosis, ability to cure has not kept pace with diagnosis, and today we behold the scientific paradox of skilled physicians sometimes knowing exactly what disease the patient is suffering from, but unable to cure the disease. In other words, *ability to diagnose, but impotence in curing*, is the true status of scientific medicine. Clinicians are floundering about in a sea of speculation and uncertainty concerning cause and cure; and the best of them declare that autopsies prove that almost half of their diagnosis are wrong.

"Every part of the body is represented by a specialist. The irony of all this professional perfection is summed up in a few words, namely, *diagnosing is an elaborate system of summing up effects without a scintilla of knowledge of cause, and the treatment is a stupendous scheme of palliation, with braggadocio concerning immunization.* But the question will not down: How is a disease to be prevented when the cause is unknown? All four hundred or more so-called diseases are nothing more than expressions of our general systemic derangement—states which I am pleased to name crises or toxemia." (The italics are mine.)

"Toxemia," as Dr. Tilden terms the degenerative condition of the blood, is principally due to a lack of alkaline elements in the blood. While the American diet is more than ample in quantity, it is deficient in alkaline elements, especially in sodium, calcium, magnesium and iron. Normal blood, containing a sufficiency of these elements supplied by natural foods, primarily fresh fruits and green-leaf vegetables grown in properly fertilized soil along with high thinking will produce in the digestive juices and secretions of the various glands, all the necessary antitoxins for the immunization of the organism. *The body will always be able to protect itself, if given the proper elements and environment for building and renewing its structure and for the proper functioning of its organs.* If this was not true, the human race could never have developed.

Why Medical Progress Is Slow

Why is it that comparatively so little progress has been made in the prevention and cure of disease since the days of Hippocrates? Merely because new, commonsense ideas were seldom accepted and taught in medical schools. Even now any teacher who tries to introduce his own ideas in opposition to those promulgated in the accepted text-books, will have difficulty in retaining his position. When Harvey discovered the circulation of the blood, most physicians and teachers over forty years of age refused to credit the discovery. It was only the younger and more independent thinkers who welcomed and understood the new theory. The adult mind, ingrained with error, often becomes fossilized and ceases to assimilate any innovation, no matter how reasonable it may be.

A rational system of healing must be constructed upon the eternal foundation of truth, upon the firm belief in nature's restorative power. Nature's efforts at healing may be assisted by an intelligent physician whose actions are governed by a thorough understanding of the laws of health and life. Future generations will certainly look upon vaccination and serum therapy as aberrations of the human mind and as legalized and commercialized falsehoods that were once kept alive by the ignorance and credulity of those who could not think for themselves.

The teachings of the great pioneers of Nature Cure, who have fought and are still fighting against the superstitions of the orthodox medical schools, are not yet fully appreciated. But every year thousands are losing faith in drug and serum methods of treating disease and are looking for sane and natural methods of living and healing. We should always be impressed with the fact, that whenever diseased conditions manifest themselves in the body, they are primarily the outcome of wrong habits of living and thinking. Local treatment will always at best produce only temporary relief. In order to get well and stay well and become useful members of human society, we must, first of all, correct our bad habits of thought and action, by acquiring self-control through a thorough understanding and practice of the laws of our being.

The wonderful creative force in the universe, which reveals itself in every cell, every atom and in every electron, is always active, protecting and preserving the life principle in the amoeba as well as in the highly organized being. It is the height of folly and conceit to believe that we can reverse the order of the universe and inure ourselves to disease by injecting poisons into our blood. Man's greatest enemies are within himself: his ignorance, selfishness, his greed and gluttony. The Cosmic Intelligence or Power which directs life's finer forces and which expresses itself in a mother's tender care during the first days of a child's earthly existence, will also safely guide us in our onward and upward struggles, if we comply with nature's higher laws in the spirit of love and service to mankind.

CHAPTER XVII

THE FUNCTION OF THE DUCTLESS GLANDS

There is a growing belief that the endocrine glands, or glands of internal secretion, have controlled the development of man from lower forms of life, and are now controlling his heredity. At a recent meeting of the American Association for the Advancement of Science the following formula was pronounced: "We are what our glands make us," which means if we are well and efficient, the credit is due to the glands; if we are sick and depressed, it is the fault of the glands. But none of the scientists thought it necessary to throw any light on the subject of who or what makes the glands.

All the glands of the body, be they ductless or not, are under the laws of the union of the organism. All organs have individual laws—a given amount of self control or individuality; but all are bound together by the blood and nervous system. In the light of common sense and reason the glands do not exist as separate entities acting for themselves, aside from the rest of the bodily organs. If the nervous system is normal, the glands are properly energized. If the habits of life are enervating, there will be a slowing up of secretions and excretions, causing a retention of waste products. The retained waste products reduce the alkalinity of the blood and cause overstimulation and enervation, affecting all parts of the body.

To restore normal action of the glands we cannot employ any specific remedies, so-called "gland foods" or "glandular extracts," but we must treat the organism in its entirety and abandon our enervating habits.

Our glands and organs have evolved as have our bodies according to natural laws. The glands are under the control of the subconscious mind the same as our heart and lungs; they function subconsciously. If the functioning becomes abnormal, it is because something has gone wrong with their nerve and food supply.

The normal function of all the glands and organs is necessary for healthy existence; they have the innate power of selecting from the blood, the elements required for growth and repair. Each gland and organ has an individuality all of its own, yet it is dependent on the entire organism for food and nerve energy. If the latter are supplied normally, general health will result. On the other hand if man lives in such a manner as to become enervated and toxic, all organs will suffer from lowering of energy; secretions and excretions are reduced and metabolical power is lowered.

When we therefore speak of the glands, we should always keep in mind that they are made from the blood, which builds the entire body. No doubt, interglandular reciprocity exists, but over all is a nervous system that furnishes energy for the proper function of the glands.

The main endocrines or ductless glands are: the *pineal, pituitary, thymus, thyroid, parathyroids, adrenals, gonads* and *spleen*. Glands that supply endocrines and also have ducts are: the liver, pancreas, kidneys, salivary and lymphatic glands.

The *pineal gland* lies near the center of the brain. It is not larger than a grain of wheat. It is said that it is the remnant of a third eye used by the primeval ancestors of man. This gland seems to be the balance of control for the action of light upon the pigment of the skin.

The *pituitary gland* is about the size of a pea and is located at the base of the brain behind the root of the nose in a little bony cup. The gland is composed of an anterior and posterior part. Each part has a distinct and separate function and secretion. The anterior part is necessary for the proper evolution of the sex glands, while the posterior part regulates the water balance of the body, blood pressure, tone of the gastro-intestinal tract; also has an influence on sugar and fat metabolism. It controls the mineral content of the blood.

The *thyroid gland* is found just below the larnyx and is composed of two lobes lying on either side of the wind pipe. It has a great controlling force in the growth of man's body and its sustaining power. It acts upon the growth of the inner and outer coverings of the body—skin, hair and mucous membranes. The thyroid is essentially an energy-producing organ and its action principle is thyroxin, almost pure iodine. With a deficiency of thyroid secretion life becomes slow and inactive, menal activity is arrested and sinks below normal, while goitre develops.

The *adrenal glands* are also two in number and are located just over the kidneys. They are as big as one's finger tips. Each gland is composed of a cortex or outer portion and the medullar or inner portion called the core. Adrenal secretion (adrin) energizes the muscles of the body, especially the muscles of the circulatory system and the digestive tract. The adrenals seem to get their potential energy from the thyroxin of the thyroid gland. *Adrin* supplies the base for saliva, pepsin, hydrochlorid acid, pancreatic and intestinal juices.

The *gonads* or *sex glands* of the male are the testicle and prostate gland; of the female they are the ovaries, breast and uterus. The gonads are of external and internal secretions. The ovaries produce the ovum, but they also produce an endocrine substance that vitalizes a woman and makes her feminine. The testes have as their external secretion the semen which carries the spermatozoa and which is stored in the prostate gland. The ovaries regulate the lime distribution in the female. During gestation an ample supply of foods rich in calcium and sodium is essential for the normal growth and development of the foetus.

The *thymus gland* is situated just below the thyroid gland and behind the upper chest bones. It seems to be the predominating gland of child growth before the time of puberty.

The *parathyroids* are composed of four tiny glands as large as wheat kernels located near the thyroid gland. Their chief function seems to be the control of the calcium metabolism or the lime salts of the system; also to control the steadiness of nerves and muscles. They regulate the detoxication of the body. There is always a lack of parathyroid endocrine secretion in lockjaw and epilepsy.

The *pancreas* has an enlongated shape, of pinkish color. It lies in front of the first and second lumbar vertebrae and behind the stomach. It weighs between two and three ounces, is about six inches long, two inches wide and one-half inch thick. It is a compound of lobules, joined together by connective tissue to form lobes, and the lobes united in the same manner, form the gland. The small ducts from each lobule open into the main duct which runs lengthwise through the gland. The pancreatic duct and the common bile duct usually enters by means of a common opening into the duodenum about three inches below the pylorus.

Scattered throughout the pancreas are round or ovoid bodies known as the *Islands of Langerhans.* Each island is about one-twenty-fifth inch in diameter and consists of a group of many-sided cells. Their function is to furnish the internal secretion of the pancreas.

Two secretions are formed in the pancreas. (1) The pancreatic fluid, which is one of the most important of the digestive fluids, is an external secretion and is poured into the duodenum during intestinal digestion. (2) The secretion formed by the Islands of Langerhans is an internal secretion that is absorbed by the blood and carried to the tissues. This internal secretion, called insulin, aids in the oxidation of glucose.

The *spleen* is directly beneath the diaphragm, behind and to the left of the stomach, and is covered by the peritoneum. The spleen acts in our body as an electric power station where the blood is recharged with electricity. This is effected by means of an apparently insignificant device by which the blood current is suddenly checked. As is well known, the arterial capillaries in all other parts of our body pass into those of the veins, but in the spleen the fine arterial capillaries terminate and become small sacs, which are called after their discoverer the "Malpighian corpuscles." There the circulation of the blood apparently is brought to a standstill.

We know the iron in the blood is magnetic in character. The sudden impact of the magnetic blood current upon the walls of the Malpighian corpuscles has the effect of converting its magnetism into electricity. We must, therefore, assume that minute electric discharges take place from the spherical walls of the Malphigian corpuscles into the blood.

The *liver* is one of the most important glands of the body. It is the storehouse and the clearing house of the system. It is here that the food is finally prepared for its advent in the circulatory system and where the broken down particles of the system are renovated and again made fit for use if possible. It is a gland of internal and external secretion. The external secretion is bile and is thrown by a duct into the digestive tract and the internal secretion is sent direct into the circulation.

The normal function of the glands depends on a well balanced diet, furnishing the needful alkaline elements, such as are outlined in the menus contained in the second part of this treatise. We have explained that chemical reactions of the endocrines and of their hormones are greatly enhanced by the presence of small amounts of such elements as iron, potassium, calcium, etc. which act as catalysts. These elements are found in green leaf vegetables, especially in the various kinds of seaweeds which can be obtained now in dehydrated and powdered form. They may be added in small amounts to our daily diet, as a safeguard against any possible deficiencies.

CHAPTER XVIII

THE DIETETIC TREATMENT OF COMMON DISEASES

We realize that so-called disease is primarily an effort of the inherent vital force of the body to eliminate waste matter and to restore the normal functioning of the organism. Natural foods, if properly selected and combined, equalize the body weight; they bring back both lean and obese individuals to a state of normality through increased alkalinity and the oxidizing power of the blood.

Healing Crises During Change of Diet

In adopting a frugal and rational diet, many persons experience at first physical discomfort, which frequently causes the faint-hearted experimenter to revert to his old dietetic habits. These disagreeable symptoms, which are often taken for a change for the worse, are really signs of improvement. As the blood becomes more alkaline, the toxins which have been retained in the tissues through years of wrong living, are dissolved and re-enter into the circulation of the blood-stream to be carried out through the excretory organs.

The process of house cleaning, or healing crises, are usually accompanied by loss of weight, mental depression, nervousness, etc., as the poisons re-enter the excretory channels. The waste materials and poisonous exudates which are being eliminated through the mucous membranes of the nasal passages, the throat, bronchi, stomach, bowels or genito-urinary organs, cause irritation and pathogenic congestion, and thus produce the well-known symptoms of inflammation and catarrhal elimination or various forms of skin eruptions. These increased processes of elimination, which are wrongly interpreted by those who do not understand nature's true healing forces, frequently frighten the patient, and cause him to return to his old way of living.

How to Permanently Relieve Constipation

Constipation is a disease of modern civilization and its many artificialities which tend to weaken our constitution. We are prone to look upon constipation as a mere local functional disorder—"The Lazy Colon," as one author expresses it. It is rather the outcome of a general state of low vitality, brought about mainly by wrong habits of living, aggravated by the strain and stress of our economic system.

The most frequent causes are lack of exercise, and the consumption of devitalized and demineralized foods which are deficient not only in cellulose, but also in the essential mineral elements, especially sodium and calcium. The latter element is indispensable for the rhythmic contraction and expansion of the muscles. A deficiency of calcium in our food is responsible for lowered tonicity of our abdominal muscles, which eventually leads to chronic intestinal stasis. It is estimated that about 75 per cent of the American people are afflicted with this condition, and it is deplorable that they seek only temporary relief by means of all kinds of more or less harmful and harmless laxatives, instead of earnestly striving to reform their dietetic habits, as well as to control their emotions and to improve the quality of their thoughts and motives.

The menus outlined in this book furnish not only a sufficiency of bulk, but also the essential alkaline salts which strengthen the abdominal muscles, and which assist in bringing about more normal and regular movements of the bowels. In the case of chronic constipation, however, quick relief is frequently necessary until the system is sufficiently strengthened, and until the bowels act of their own accord.

Under such conditions, mildly laxative herbal teas and preparations, emanating from trustworthy sources, and rich in blood-purifying, non-griping herbs will prove non-injurious and beneficial. A natural intestinal lubricant is provided in *Plantago Psyllium Seed;* unlike mineral oil and its by-products, it is not inorganic and serves the double purpose of providing bulk and lubrication. Agar-Agar, made from a Japanese seaweed, stimulates the bowels in a mechanical way. Through its ability to absorb water, Agar-Agar expands to ten times its original bulk, forming in the colon a bland, bulky mass. This swollen soft and moist material, while not absorbed by the system, mixes with the food intake and subsequently becomes a constituent of the stool, modifying and softening its consistency.

The Cause of Heart Failure and Apoplexy

Two serious diseases that are rapidly increasing are heart failure and apoplexy—the results of fast living, overpowering fears and anxieties, and aggravated by the extensive use of meat, coffee, tea, alcoholic beverages and tobacco. These habits are characteristic of our commercial age, reflecting our greed and selfishness, where the quick accumulation of a fortune is the prime object in life. In their wild chase after elusive wealth and in their neglect of hygienic laws, people constantly must have recourse to stimulants. Heart failure generally occurs in connection with arteriosclerosis, high blood pressure, diabetes, gout, and with kindred afflictions. A man is as old as his arteries, because the circulation of the blood depends upon the arterial tension. The heart alone could not perform the tremendous task of forcing the blood continually through the arteries and capillaries were it not for the arteries themselves by means of which their muscular walls assist in circulating the blood. If through constant overeating and over-stimulation, the arterial walls gradually become encumbered with phosphates, urates and with other waste matter and thereby narrow the openings of the blood vessels and deprive them of their natural muscular elasticity, additional work is thrown upon the heart. The constantly increasing blood pressure, inevitably resulting, often causes fatal hemorrhages. Every day we see men in the prime of life suddenly succumb to apoplexy and paralysis, due to abnormal blood pressure, resulting from the accumulation of waste matter in the system and of consequent hardening of the arteries.

Cancer, Its Cause and Prevention

Another disease which is on the increase is cancer. New and fantastic cures for it are discovered and proclaimed almost monthly. The proportion of cancer cases in a community likewise appears to be in direct ratio to its consumption of meat, salt, sugar, spices, coffee, tobacco and alcohol. There is no doubt that the cause of all malignant growths of the body is a highly toxic condition of the blood, the result of years of irrational living and thinking. Not all abnormal enlargements of the tissues are of a cancerous character, and in the majority of cases a strictly regulated, simple diet will reduce abnormal tissue formations. There are no cancer cures except the alkaline elements of a diet consisting largely of fresh fruits and vegetables, combined with natural therapeutic measures which assist in the elimination of waste matter. It is also imperative that we raise our mental and psychic vibrations to higher altitudes of thought, will and feeling. Surgical operations never strike at the root of the evil and only temporarily remove the symptoms of the disease.

Loss of Weight Due to Faulty Digestion

Underweight or emaciation is due to a low state of vitality and to the inability of the individual to properly digest and assimilate his food. The causes of such faulty digestion and assimilation are the eating of devitalized foods, the drug habit, worry, fear, excesses of all kinds, loss of sleep, etc., which interfere with the proper functioning of the gastro-intestinal nerves and with the formation of the glandular secretions, constantly involving a large expenditure of nerve force.

We find these conditions in nearly all cases of chronic catarrh and tuberculosis, which have been treated with so-called nourishing foods. It is folly to prescribe for such people large quantities of milk, eggs and meat which but further encumber the system with waste matter. At all times the diet should be adapted to the digestive and assimilative power of the patient. A diet consisting largely of fresh fruits, fruit juices and vegetables properly prepared will soon improve the quality of the blood and increase the strength of the digestive juices, thus gradually working towards better assimilation and normal tissue-building.

DIABETES MELLITUS

Diabetes, a disease resulting criefly from faulty nutrition and uncontrolled emotions, is also steadily on the increase. The characteristic symptoms of this disease are obesity and the abnormal sugar content of the blood, frequently over 0.3 per cent, which is three or four times more than is normal. As a result of the large consumption of meat, sugar and white flour products, diabetes has become a common disease in the United States. We must not regard diabetes as a mere local disturbance in the function of the pancreas, but as a sign of physical degeneration due to a highly acid-forming diet. Diabetes is essentially a disease of physical degeneration due to a highly acid forming diet, lack of exercise and unbridled psychic impulses.

There are two forms of diabetes, one is called *Diabetes Mellitus,* which is characterized by a greater or less amount of sugar, and the other form is called *Diabetes Insipidus,* where the urine is as great in quantity and in frequency, but contains no sugar or any other abnormal ingredients. It is the sugar form of the disease, the type that is called Diabetes Mellitus or Glycosuria, that is the more serious and important ailment.

Until about forty years ago it was thought that diabetes was a symptom vaguely associated with diseases of the liver and kidneys, and with many other conditions, but during the last twenty-five or thirty years the disease has been attributed to disturbances of a degenerate kind in the pancreas, and more particularly of late, of certain specific areas of the pancreas called the Islands of Langerhans, which secrete the so-called insulin, essential for the digestion of sugar.

Insulin—A Will o' the Wisp

Insulin, now employed, is a fluidic remedy injected directly into the blood stream and is supposed to have a beneficial effect upon diabetic patients. It is extracted from certain parts of the pancreas, a gland located in back of and slightly below the stomach. When this gland is removed from the animal and used as food, it is called sweetbread.

The word insulin is used to describe this fluid because the parts of the pancreas from which it is extracted exist in small bunches of cells, grouped together like little islands, and hence known as the *"Islands of Langerhans."* The remaining parts of the pancreas consist of tissues which produce liquid enzymes and ferments and which flow through a duct into the first part of the duodenum just outside of the pyloric opening of the stomach, where they mix with the gastric secretions and aid in the digestion of food. In making insulin these parts of the pancreatic gland are excluded and only the so-called "Islands of Langerhans" are used. However this may be, the only difference between the work of Doctor Banting, who is the accredited discoverer of insulin, and that of earlier investigators consists in Doctor Banting's separation of the two.

Many medical men now admit that up to the present, insulin can do nothing more than to relieve only temporarily the incurable defect of sugar storage after each injection, and careful and cautious doctors are gradually discontinuing the use of this dangerous nostrum. In fact, in certain institutions and hospitals throughout the world, the use of insulin has been completely abandoned and diabetic patients are now being treated by diet alone, without ever resorting to insulin or even referring to it.

There is some evidence for believing that diabetes is hereditary for it is found to attack several members of a family simultaneously and consecutively. Careful investigations prove that hereditary tendencies, when they show themselves in any families, are the result of similar dietetic habits, along with similar living conditions and circumstances. The great prevalence of the disease in our modern towns and large cities, where one hundred pounds of refined sugar per capita are consumed yearly as compared with ten pounds per capita consumed twenty-five years ago, is another proof that hereditary causes are extremely subordinate; that they can be intelligently combatted and their influence mitigated. When we add to these predisposing causes the additional fact that almost everybody living nowadays eats an excess of meat, concentrated sweets and starchy foods, we must conclude that the excessive use of these foods is in some way or another the direct cause of Diabetes Mellitus, and that other causes are only secondary or predisposing.

Dr. Rasmus Alsaker, a physician of wide experience, gives the following excellent advice in his *"Monthly Health Review"*:

"We know from our own experience that the diabetics are leaning too heavily on insulin. Surely you know that insulin cures nothing. It does not help the patient to build a better blood stream and it does not help him to improve his general health. It often lulls him into a false sense of security so that he does nothing for himself. If a person with diabetes takes insulin and continues to live in the same old way, he will not live as long as he could. He will continue to grow more and more acid and his body will deteriorate from year to year until nothing more can be done for him. We have seen chronic insulin takers so anemic that they appeared to be made from wax, showing no color in the lips and very pale mucous membrane in the mouth. This is a dangerous state of affairs.

"Insulin does just one thing and that is to help burn the sugar produced from the digestion of one meal. Its effect is not noticeable more than a few hours. Then another dose of insulin has to be taken, with the body deteriorating all the time. We may repeat, but we think we are justified because many persons look upon insulin as a cure for diabetes when in truth it is only a palliative for a few hours. We would urge those readers who happen to be afflcted in this way not to lean on insulin. If they are using it now they should strive to reduce the dose and build up the general health through judicious living. We shall outline how this is done.

"1. See to it that the elimination is excellent. We talk so much about the elimination that it may bore some of the old subscibers, but please be forbearing and remember that new subscribers are coming to us every month. The four great eliminating organs are the skin, the lungs, the kidneys and the bowels. We have just been explaining that with proper food and drink the kidneys will care for themselves. Diabetics should drink at least eight glasses, or sixty-four ounces, of water every day. They should see to it that the bowels move freely twice a day, or at the very least once a day. They should practice deep breathing until it is established as a habit. They should apply friction to the entire surface of the body once or twice every day.

"2. They should be in the open air as much as possible during good weather and they should ventilate thoroughly at night.

"3. They should not attempt any violent exercise, but they should take enough walking and exercise for the rest of the body to maintain a lively circulation.

"4. In diabetes the body is very toxic and the patient should not add to the poisons in his body by consuming tobacco, coffee, tea and alcohol. Water is the best drink for them and for everybody else.

"5. The eating must be balanced. It is very essential not to give a person with diabetes excessive amounts of starches and sweets. We know that some professional men tell their patients to eat any old thing and take a dose of insulin and forget about it, but this is a very serious error.

"Our experience has been that diabetics can take care of some starch, but that all starch does not react alike. We get much better results with baked potatoes than we do with whole wheat bread in diabetes. It is almost impossible to lay out a general diet for those suffering from diabetes because each case differs from all the rest. It is an individual proposition, but we shall attempt something that we know will be far better than the hit and miss plan of the majority. We are in the habit of recommending nuts in this ailment. They are easy to digest if thoroughly masticated and they do not contain enough starch to be objectionable, with the exception of the chestnut, which is barred. Of course, we do not recommend peanuts, but they are legumes and not nuts.

"It is true that all fruits contain some sugar, but those that are low in sugar content can be used to good advantage, among them apples, pears and a moderate amount of grapefruit. We would advise that these patients avoid such sugary fruits as grapes, raisins, figs, dates, prunes and thoroughly ripe bananas until the diabetes is under control. After that some of these foods may be used in moderation. We remember one of our patients who had an extreme case of diabetes. At first we took away from him all foods containing sugar and starch to exceed six per cent, but after he recovered he was able to eat potatoes, prunes, and nearly all the fruits without any difficulty.

At first it is best to leave out of the feeding plan such starchy vegetables as parsnips, beets, peas, lima beans, butterbeans and carrots. Perhaps we should have called the beets a sugary vegetable, for it is the sugar in them that is objectionable. After recovery is made these vegetables may be used with discretion. Some of the permitted vegetables are Swiss chard, spinach, lettuce, celery, cucumbers, tomatoes, romaine, endive, cabbage, cauliflower, turnips, asparagus, onions, string beans and all other leafy vegetables that you can find in the market or in your garden. Tender young beet tops and turnip tops are excellent.

"Diabetics usually eat more meat than is good for them. Please remember that an excess of meat causes an acid body and that is a handicap in recovering. We have made a practice of continuing the meat eating to one meal and permitting nuts in one or two meals. Nuts are far more nourishing than meat or bread and they really take the place of both, for they are rich in oil and protein."

The following report is from the New York Times:

"Despite the widespread use of insulin, in treating diabetics during the last ten years, this disease claimed four times as many victims in New York City last year as it did thirty years ago, according to a survey made by public officials of the New York Tuberculosis and Health Association.

The survey recently was completed by Godias J. Drolet, statistician for the New York Tuberculosis and Health Association, for the organization's research service. The actual figures show that 2,116 died from diabetes in 1932, compared with 503 deaths in 1901, a rise from fourteen deaths per 100,000 population to twenty-nine per 100,000.

"This increase," Mr. Drolet explained, "has been almost wholly confined to women. In 1901 the 503 deaths were fairly equally divided between the sexes with 269 deaths among males and 234 among females. In 1931 a total of 633 men and 1,288 women died of diabetes."

In explaining this increase, Mr. Drolet said: "When the city's population doubled that of 1901, the deaths from diabetes numbered four times as many and the mortality of the female sex became twice that among the males. In my opinion this increase among women is probably due to the noticeable release from physical labor and home drudgery, lightened by the 'machine age' that the so-called modern woman of America enjoys. Diabetes is possibly a concomitant of reduced physical exercise—throwing a greater load on the internal organs."

To evaluate properly the increase in diabetic deaths, special studies of the change in population were made. Not only the increase in population, but the change in the age grouping was accounted for, and standardized rates for each year of the thirty year period under scrutiny were prepared.

While the crude death rate from diabetes per 100,000 population rose from 14.2 in 1901 to 27.1 in 1931, or nearly doubled, the standardized rate, taking into account growth and adjusted for comparison on the basis of a similar age composition, changed from 17.3 to 27.9, or truly rose by 58 per cent.

"Insulin, already at our disposal for more than ten years," said Mr. Drolet, "does not seem to be sufficiently effective in checking this rise. Although it has undoubtedly prolonged the life of many diabetic sufferers, it is obvious that greater efforts must be made on the preventive side. Insulin can only relieve the condition among those already suffering from diabetes. We must ascertain the true cause leading to this disease."

There are no specific foods or remedies necessary to cure diabetes, except a carefully selected diet of fruits and vegetables, supplying the needful alkaline elements to eliminate the toxins from the system. The widely advertised gluten products and other "diabetic" foods are worse than useless because they are acid forming. Saccharine, a coal tar product, is often used by diabetics in place of sugar, but in every instance the drug will prove harmful to the patient, as it will affect the normal function of the kidneys.

The Fruit and Absolute Fast

Complete abstinence from food one day each week will greatly assist the eliminative organs to restore normal function. An occasional fruit fast, which means living exclusively on fresh fruits, for one or two weeks, will also be found most effective in loosening and dissolving the morbid matter in the body. An absolute fast is best taken under the direction of a competent nature cure physician, and should always be preceded by an exclusive fruit diet of one or two weeks' duration. Since Dr. Henry S. Tanner undertook his famous forty-two day fast in 1877, fasting has been recognized as one of the most effective therapeutic measures. During the last twenty-five years, hundreds of people have fasted from one to seven weeks under medical supervision. In most instances the fast resulted in improved health and enabled the patient to regain normal weight rapidly. Whenever death occurred during the fast, it was caused by organic defects which were beyond repair. It is, however, the consensus of opinion among many close observers that prolonged fasts should not be taken by people of a nervous or emotional temperament, especially by those who are below normal in weight. It often requires years of careful living to overcome the shock received by the nervous system from an injudiciously long fast. But in cases of fever and inflammation, fasting for one or two weeks is essential for quick recovery. It gives the organs of digestion a much needed rest, so that the organism can concentrate its nerve force on the elimination of waste poisons. A long fast is best broken by sipping small quantities of fruit juices or vegetable broths at intervals of several hours during the first two days, in order to gradually restore the digestive organs to their normal functions.

We should possess the understanding that the body is an organic whole; that in the last analysis all diseases have one common origin—diminished vital force or enervation—whether caused by auto-intoxication or drug and serum medication, and that while restoring normal and healthy conditions, the organism has to pass through a series of healing crises during which these poisons are eliminated. Successful treatment, therefore, cannot consist in confining one's efforts to the organ or part affected, but the organism must be treated in its entirety. In adopting a rational diet, by means of which the blood is gradually purified, we cannot expect an immediate restoration of health. The blood has to be first restored to its normal alkalinity, and all encumbrances eliminated to ensure perfect circulation of the blood. This may often take months or even years, but this should not discourage those who want to achieve lasting health.

PART II

PRACTICAL DIETETICS

CHAPTER XIX

THE RATIONAL PREPARATION OF FOODS

In the present chapter and the succeeding one the author shall try to simplify as much as possible the correct preparation and combination of foods, and to provide, in a comparatively small amount of nourishment, a sufficiency of all the essential food elements for maintaining health and vitality. We have shown in the preceding pages that this can be accomplished by eating mostly natural, uncooked foods in which the alkaline elements predominate. If the blood is daily supplied with the right quantity and proportion of wholesome fruits and green-leaf vegetables, it will contain a much larger amount of the alkaline bases than it does of acids. *And it is only when the blood has a normal alkaline reaction that our organs of digestion and assimilation and our glands can function normally, thus completely neutralizing and eliminating waste matter and toxins and maintaining bodily heat and electricity.* If they are surrounded by strongly alkaline fluids, the cells of the body are preserved better and need less frequent replacement. The rigors of a northern climate, as well as tropical heat and sudden changes in temperature can always be borne with hardly any inconvenience when the blood is free from toxins and its circulation is not obstructed.

The Importance of an Alkaline Diet

If the alkalinity of the blood is diminished by the constant use of wrong foods, all the processes of digestion and elimination are retarded. The acids of the blood will attack the bones and muscular tissues and deprive them of their alkaline bases, in order to neutralize as much as possible the constantly forming toxins.

Thus we see with an acid-forming diet, in which meat, refined sugar and cereal foods predominate, a larger amount of protein is necessary to replace the abnormally daily loss and to maintain the nitrogen equilibrium of the body than with a diet which contains a sufficiency of fresh or dried fruits and green-leaf vegetables. On account of their high alkalinity the latter may be called tissue-protecting foods. A high protein diet further increases the acidity of the blood and seriously impairs the organs of digestion and elimination by constantly overtaxing them.

Chemical analysis shows that green-leaf vegetables contain from 1 to 3.5 per cent of protein of the highest order, fresh fruits from 0.5 to 2.5 per cent, and nuts from 5 to 30 per cent. This protein is formed directly, by means of the sunlight in the protoplasmic cells of the plant. It is, therefore, much superior in the building and reconstructive processes of the body to that contained in the more or less worn-out cells of meat, in which the vibratory forces of life are descensive. Only from 1 to 1½ ounces of protein (30 to 45 grams), in the form of nuts, nut-butters, legumes, or dairy products, combined with fresh fruit and vegetables, are required for a well-balanced daily dietary under normal conditions. For instance, 4 ounces of nuts or fresh cottage cheese amply supplies the average daily protein requirements of most adults.

"Meat Substitutes" Not Essential

Those persons who want to adopt a meatless diet should not look for artifically prepared meat substitutes as a source of protein. A food constituent required in such a limited amount as is protein is easily supplied by the various products of the vegetable kingdom. Such combinations as "roast vegetable turkey" or "vegetarian steak" seem to be the result of the belief that meat is a necessary food and must be replaced in some form. Indeed, vegetarians who live largely on foods in which the protoplasmic cells have been more or less disorganized by prolonged cooking have very little advantage over mixed eaters.

All other factors being equal, a judiciously selected meatless diet is far more conducive to health than is the usual mixed diet, consisting, for the most part, of animal and starch-bearing foods deficient in alkaline elements. We should understand that the proteins of fruits and vegetables, supplanted by a small amount of the proteins of nuts, legumes (especially soy beans), or dairy products are fully able to maintain health and efficiency. It is entirely feasible to live on an exclusive diet of fresh ripe fruits and green-leaf vegetables for many weeks and months, thereby purifying the blood and greatly improving the keenness of our senses. In fact, in many pathological conditions such a restricted diet is more helpful than is an absolute fast.

Among the legumes which contain a large amount of protein, the *soy bean* takes first place. Its protein content, nearly 40%, is higher than that of any other food. Moreover, this protein is of excellent quality, as valuable as is the casein of milk; it contains all the essential animo acids. It embodies a sufficiency of vitamins A and B, and in this respect it is superior to all seeds. Very little carbohydrate enters into its composition, only about 6%, and it is practically free from starch. The soy bean fills the place of meat as well as that of milk in the dietary of many millions of sturdy Orientals; it is destined to become one of the great food staples, not only of this country, but of the world. A number of recipes for the preparation of the soy bean are given in this chapter.

Wastefulness of Food Preparation

A great deal of time and money is wasted in the usual methods of preparing food for the table. It is said that the American housewife is the most extravagant in the world. This extravagance consists chiefly in buying and serving more food than is necessary, in irrational preparation and in throwing away many nourishing portions, especially the water in which the vegetables have been cooked. Thousands of cook-books have been written, vegetarian and otherwise, containing recipes of the most incompatible mixtures of foods and condiments. We often find sugar, salt, pepper, baking powder in a single recipe, while acid fruits are frequently mixed with cornstarch and refined sugar. Some of the menus are made up of a dozen or more different dishes. Probably only half of the food set on the table is consumed, while the other half goes into the garbage can. This waste occurs not only in hotels and in the mansions of the well-to-do, but also in many homes of clerks and workingmen. In fact, the waste of food in the United States each year is estimated to be over $700,000,000. It is the daily loss of small quantities of food in thousands of homes and restaurants that brings the total to such enormous proportions. The loss of time and money through impaired health caused by this extravagant eating, probably is much larger.

The housewife often prides herself on the preparation of sumptuous dinners, forgetting that in most instances she can hardly improve on the natural qualities and flavor of the foods. The display of a great variety of dishes leads to overeating. An argument of the greatest importance for a simple and natural diet —especially from the economic and social point of view—is that such a diet means the emancipation of woman from kitchen slavery. She can then utilize the time which she formerly devoted to cooking, baking, frying (and their resulting ailments), to the proper education of her children and to her own cultural advancement.

FRUITS, DRIED AND CANNED, AND FRUIT JUICES

Fruits need the least preparation of all foods. They can be eaten just as we receive them from nature, unblemished by the hand of man. Many fruits such as berries, grapes, apples, apricots, pears, peaches, figs, etc. can be eaten with the skins after they have been thoroughly cleansed. As the season for fresh fruit is comparatively short, various ways have been devised to preserve the surplus for the winter months. The best methods are: preservation of the juice, canning, dehydration and sun-drying.

Dried fruits are more wholesome and economical than are canned fruits. The difference between canned fruits and dried fruits, both in regard to price and hygienic value, is seldom realized. For instance, a can of apricots retailing at 25 cents contains one pound of fruit and twelve ounces of cane syrup manufactured from refined sugar. One pound of the best evaporated apricots requires nearly seven pounds of fresh fruit and retails for about 50 cents. It therefore furnishes almost as much real food value as do seven cans of apricots. The syrup, being devoid of organic salts, is used only as a preservative. The consumer has to pay for the cost of the syrup and canning, also for the increased cost of transportation and warehousing.

The injuriousness of bleaching fruits with sulphurous acid before the drying process has been pointed out. We should therefore be careful to use only unsulphured fruits, especially for children and convalescents. The detrimental effects of sulphurous acid upon the system may not be immediately noticed, but they will certainly make themselves felt in the course of time. The methods of dehydrating fruits have been very much improved during the last ten years and unsulphured dried fruits can now be produced with but a little more expense than is the case with sulphured fruits, although the latter may be lighter in color and more attractive to the eye.

Dried fruits can be made almost like fresh fruits by the following method: Place the desired quantity of dried fruit in a dish and add enough soft or distilled water to cover them. After standing from 16 to 20 hours the fruit will have absorbed sufficient moisture and may then be slightly heated to about 100 degrees Fahrenheit, if desired. Dried fruits should never be boiled as they lose a good deal of their natural flavor by excessive heat. The water in which the fruit was soaked makes a delicious food drink. The fruits best adapted for making fresh fruit juices in the home are oranges, grapes and berries.

The Preserving of Fruit Juices

Fruit juice can be preserved by heating it to about 170 degrees Fahrenheit in enameled kettles, and then filling it in jars or bottles which have been kept in hot water. The receptacles are then hermetically sealed. Bottles made for crown corks, which can easily be attached by a small hand-machine, are best adapted for this purpose. In order to destroy all yeast and mould germs. it is necessary to put the filled bottles into a suitable metal tank with hot water, kept at a consistent temperature of 175 degrees Fahrenheit for about 40 mintues.

The usual methods of canning fruits with the addition of refined sugar should not be encouraged. Honey diluted with two parts water should be substituted. Many fruits can be preserved without the addition of any sweetening. Whenever possible, drying or dehydrating fruits and vegetables should be employed instead of canning.

Those persons desiring specific information on these subjects should write to the United States Department of Agriculture. Washington, D. C., for the following bulletins which are distributed free of charge:

Farmers' Bulletin No. 900 "Home-made Fruit Butters."
Farmers' Bulletin No. 984 "Farm and Home Drying of Fruits and Vegetables."
Farmers' Bulletin No. 1,075 "Unfermented Grape Juice: How to Make It in the Home."
Farmers' Bulletin No. 1,211 "Home Canning of Fruits and Vegetables."
Farmers' Bulletin No. 1,264 "Farm Manufacture of Unfermented Apple Juice."

Oily Fruits

Fruits, with the exception of the olive and avocado, contain very little fat The ripe olive has about 20 per cent fat; 100 pounds of olives are necessary to make 3 gallons of oil—that is, if hydraulic presses are used to extract the oil from the macerated pulp. Olive oil is undoubtedly one of the best oils for human consumption. It is a highly concentrated food principle, consisting of nearly

100 per cent fat. It should, therefore, be used sparingly, preferably in combination with vegetable salads. In southern Europe dried olives are a popular food. They lose some of their bitter taste during the ripening and drying process and are generally eaten together with bread, dried fruits and salad vegetables. The fat in the dried olive exists in a state of emulsion and is organically combined with protein and mineral salts, which are lacking in the canned and pickled olive. Such olives are usually treated in several lye solutions which wash out most of the essential ingredients. A palatable combination of pitted dried olives and prunes is suggested as a spread or filling and as a laxative prune dessert.

The avocado is a tropical fruit but it can be successfully grown in subtropical countries like Southern California and Florida. Avocados grow on beautiful evergreen trees and the hardier varieties stand as much frost as does the orange tree. The weight of the fruit varies from a few ounces to 1 pound and more. Its smooth and buttery consistency and rich nutty flavor distinguish it from all other fruits. It contains on an average 2 per cent protein, while the best varieties have more than 20 per cent fat in a very palatable and digestible form. The mineral matter shows a preponderance of the alkaline elements. Avocados make an excellent addition to combination salads.

FRUIT AND NUT CONFECTIONS

Fruit and nut confections made without refined sugar should take the place of candies, which are placed in ever changing forms and names before the American public. Sweetmeats prepared from nuts and unsulphured fruits without refined sugar present a fine confection for growing children, who have a natural craving for sweets. The pernicious influence of artificial refined sweets upon the teeth and digestive organs has been pointed out repeatedly in the preceding chapters.

Fruit and nut confections which can be made in endless varieties and shapes are concentrated foods which, when eaten together with some fresh fruits, such as apples, bananas, oranges, etc. make a complete and satisfying lunch; they are also an ideal diet for travelers, as a few days' supply can be conveniently carried along. Fresh fruits such as apples, bananas and oranges can now be procured most everywhere during all seasons of the year. The traveler does not have to depend on quick lunch counters for his food supply, if he has provided himself with a few pounds of natural sweetmeats. To the long distance walker and mountain climber the various preparations of fruits and nuts are a wonderful help, as they furnish in a compact form the wholesome natural sugars and fats for producing muscular energy and increasing endurance. Fatigue is considerably lessened with a fruit and nut diet, as the production of waste poisons is reduced, while their elimination is promoted by the alkaline salts of the fruits. It is a well known fact that meat greatly lessens endurance, as it increases the formation of toxins in the muscular tissues.

STUFFED DATES

Remove the pit by opening the side of the date with a pointed knife and insert a pecan or blanched almond.

STUFFED PRUNES

Steam large size prunes in order to soften the meat and loosen the pit. which can be removed in the same way as with the date. Insert half walnuts or large blanched almonds. Almond butter mixed with a little grated cocoanut may be used in place of the nuts.

DATE CARAMELS*

2 pounds pitted dates
½ pound blanched almonds
½ pound shelled walnuts or pignolias

If necessary a cup of flaked cereals can be added to give the mixture the proper consistency. Mix the ingredients and run through a food chopper twice in order to get the mixture perfectly smooth. Press into a flat pan in a layer of about ¾ inch thickness and let stand for a few hours. The pan should be laid out with heavy wax paper, so the contents can be removed easily on a board. Cut into ¾ inch cubes by means of a sharp knife. Seedless raisins, blanched peanuts and grated cocoanuts may be substituted for dates, almonds and walnuts.

NUT FRUITOSE*

1 cup pitted dates
1 cup figs (stems should be cut off)
1 cup seedless raisins
½ cup almond meats
½ cup walnuts or filbert meats

Mix the ingredients and run through the food chopper twice. Press the mixture into a flat pan in a layer about 1 inch thick, let stand overnight and cut into convenient sizes.

CAROB CONFECTION

½ pound carob meal
½ pound seedless raisins
½ pound pitted dates
1 cup flaked cereals, or macaroon cocoanut in order to give the mixture the right consistency.

Run through the chopper twice in order to thoroughly blend the ingredients. Press into a pan and let it stand overnight. Cut into convenient sizes.

RAISIN-NUT BALLS*

1 cup shelled Brazil nuts
1 cup shelled pecans
1 cup shelled walnuts
2 cups seedless raisins
½ cup grated cocoanut
2 tablespoons honey

Run the nuts and raisins through the food chopper first separately, then together with the honey, in order to thoroughly blend the ingredients into a homogeneous mixture. Form into balls of about ¾ inch in diameter and roll into the grated cocoanut, to give them an attractive appearance.

RAISIN COCOANUT CARAMELS

2 cups seedless raisins
2 cups grated cocoanut

Mix and run through the food chopper several times, in order to thoroughly blend the ingredients. Roll out on a board about ½ inch thick and cut into squares. For a change 2 cups of pitted and chopped dates can be used instead of raisins.

**One kind of nut is best where stomach is weak and digestion not up to par.

HONEY COCOANUT BALLS

2 cups grated cocoanut
½ cup strained honey

Thoroughly mix the honey with the cocoanut until it is a homogeneous mixture. Form into balls about ¾ inch thick and top them with a pecan nut.

As already mentioned, many varieties of fruit and nut confections can be made by using different kinds of unsulphured dried fruits and grinding them together in various proportions and shaping them into such forms as will suit individual taste and fancy.

NUTS AND NUT BUTTER

Nuts do not constitute a very large part of the dietary of civilized man simply because their cultivation has been neglected and little has been known of their high nutritive value. A great deal has been said of the indigestibility of nuts. But this may be attributed largely to the fact that, as a general rule, they are either eaten on top of a heavy meal or else insufficiently masticated. Until quite recently almonds, English walnuts, pecans and many of the imported nuts have been merely considered a luxury, to be used only on special occasions, as table decoration for the holidays.

Nuts are nature's most concentrated foods and their high nutritive value, in comparison with that of animal foods, is becoming more widely recognized. Nuts contain very little starch, except the chestnut which has 70 per cent. The average amount does not exceed 10 per cent. The almond contains a negligible amount of starch, but has 6 per cent sugar. This makes it invaluable in the preparation of infant foods.

The fat in nuts, which averages 50 per cent, is much more easily digested than is animal fat, such as lard, tallow and butter. Animal fat is a free fat and will not mix with water, while the fat of nuts mixes freely with water and forms an emulsion resembling cream.

The digestion and assimilation of fats depend on the constant supply of organic sodium in our food. Sodium is the principal alkaline element in the process of saponification which is carried on by the pancreatic juice, the bile and the intestinal juice. The proper functioning of the latter depends on its content of carbonate of soda. This is essential for the neutralization of the acids of the intestinal tract as well as for the emulsification of the fats. The digestibility of nuts is always greatly increased by eating them together with vegetables and fruits, which are rich in sodium (see table in the appendix of this volume, giving amount of sodium in foods), but not by the addition of coarse table salt As a matter of fact, salting and roasting greatly impair the nutritive value of nuts and prevent their proper assimilation. The proteins become coagulated by roasting, and the fats split into glycerine and free fatty acids, while the vitamins are destroyed. Nut butters made from salted nuts should, therefore, have no place in our dietary.

Since few people, on account of defective teeth, can masticate nuts well enough to be acted upon by the digestive juices, the mechanical emulsification of nuts by means of nut butter mills is quite indispensable.

Peanuts, almonds and cashew nuts are used chiefly for this purpose, but brazil nuts, pignolias, filberts and walnuts also make fine butters, although some of these nuts cannot be blanched very easily. The blanching of peanuts and almonds is now done on a large scale by special machinery, and the blanched nuts can be procured in nearly all the larger cities. The nuts should be broken into small pieces by running them through a loosely adjusted food chopper. The pieces should be put into a moderately hot oven for a few minutes to make them dry and crisp before they are run through the tightly adjusted nut mill. Care should be taken not to have the nuts too brown or scorched; they should simply be as crisp as possible, for in this condition they make smooth and palatable nut butter. If the nuts are too moist, they will form a stiff paste and clog the mill.

To blanch peanuts in small quantities, heat them slightly and then spread on a table and lightly press them with a rolling-pin. This will loosen the skins sufficiently to enable one to blow them away. Unroasted peanut butter is more healthful and digestible than is the roasted kind.

To blanch almonds, soak them in boiling water for about three minutes. The skins then become loose and can be pinched off by pressing the nuts with the thumb and first finger. The almonds, of course, become moist in this process and they should be put into a moderately hot oven for a few minutes. To facilitate the drying, the almonds are best ground into a coarse meal by means of a food chopper. Brazil nuts, which can be bought shelled, need not be blanched but they are best broken into small pieces by means of a food chopper before running them through the nut mill.

Pignolias, which are imported from Italy and Spain, are already shelled and blanched and can be used for making nut butter without further preparation except washing and drying in a moderately hot oven.

Cocoanuts can be bought either shredded or granulated. They are dessicated and packed in the countries in which they are grown, principally in Ceylon and the Philippine Islands. Grated or shredded cocoanuts, if free from moisture, can be ground into nut butter. Whole cocoanuts can frequently be procured at the fruitstands of larger cities, but it needs some practice to shell them without breaking the nuts into small pieces.

COCOANUT MILK

2 cups boiling water
1 cup grated cocoanut

Thoroughly beat and work together for 10 minutes. Then pass the mixture through a clean cheese cloth. The cocoanut may be used in the same way a second time in order to extract all milk.

COMBINATION NUT BUTTER

Grind equal parts of peanuts (blanched), pignolias and grated cocoanuts through a nut mill. The nuts should be heated slightly before grinding to remove as much as possible of the moisture, in order to make a smooth butter.

NUT CREAM (Nut Butter Dressing)

To make a very palatable nut cream, first dissolve the desired quantity of unroasted nut butter in a little warm water so as to make a very fine paste, afterwards adding warm water enough to bring the cream to the proper consistency. Keep in a cool place. It is best not to make any more nut cream than will be used during the day. This cream may be used instead of dairy cream for ordinary purposes with excellent results. The addition of a little honey enhances its flavor. About 2 tablespoons nut butter will make 1 cup nut butter dressing.

NUT MILK

Nut milk is made by adding more water to the nut cream. The further addition of a little honey or sweet fruit juice makes this milk very palatable. It should be sipped slowly and insalivated thoroughly in order to insure good digestion. Unroasted almond butter is best for making nut milk for children.

NUT MEAL

Grind the different nuts through a loosely adjusted nut mill. This nut meal may also be used for baking purposes and for various kinds of fruit and nut confections, also for sprinkling over fruit and vegetable salads.

NUT CREAM CUSTARD

3 eggs
1 teaspoon honey
2 cups nut milk
Flavoring

Beat eggs, add honey and flavoring (vanilla, lemon or chocolate, etc.), then add nut cream and beat the whole again. Pour in custard dishes and steam until knife comes out clean. Be careful not to cook too long.

For thin custard, beat white of eggs separately, add nuts before cooking and mix it up well with the whole. Stir constantly until the custard coats the spoon, when it is done.

NUT LOAVES, ETC.

SAVORY NUT LOAF

1 cup ground cereals or bread crumbs
3 cups finely chopped vegetables
2 cups thin nut butter dressing
1 tablespoon savory herbs (marjoram, sage or savory)
1 tablespoon chopped parsley

Mix well, put into an oiled pan and bake in a moderately hot oven for about 45 minutes

SPINACH NUT LOAF

1 cup pignolias or blanched peanuts ground fine
1 bunch spinach washed and cut fine
1 onion finely chopped
1 tablespoon chopped parsley
1 cup dry, ground bread crumbs
1 egg beaten

Steam the vegetables in a waterless cooker until tender, add the nuts, egg, bread crumbs and mix all the ingredients thoroughly. Shape into a loaf, cover with cracker dust, brush with vegetable oil and bake about 25 minutes.

PEANUT LOAF

2 cups blanched peanuts, ground fine
2 cups cracker crumbs, or flaked cereals
1 cup water
2 eggs beaten
1 chopped onion, medium size
2 tablespoons whole wheat flour

Mix all the ingredients thoroughly and bake in a moderately hot oven for about 1 hour.

PECAN LOAF*

1 cup finely chopped pecans
1 cup of a preferred protein flour or meal, or a flaked soya bean cereal.
1 tablespoon chopped parsley
1 egg

Mix together pecans, preferred protein meal or flaked soy cereal and parsley. Beat the egg and mix with the other ingredients. Mold into a loaf and bake slowly for 45 minutes.

PIGNOLIA LOAF

1 cup pignolias ground fine
½ cup Brazil nuts ground fine
2 cups bread crumbs or flaked soy cereal
1 cup water
2 tablespoons nut butter dressing
1 tablespoon chopped parsley
1 onion chopped fine
½ teaspoon sage

Mix all the ingredients and form into one or two loaves. Put into oiled pans and bake in a moderate oven for ¾ hour.

WALNUT PATTIES

1 cup ground walnuts
2 cups of a preferred protein flour or meal
1 grated carrot, medium size
1 onion chopped fine
2 eggs beaten
2 cups strained tomato pulp

Mix together the first four items and form into small patties. Cover with the tomato pulp and bake 20 minutes.

---

*Some dietitians do not recommend gluten flour as a protein filler since it contains on the average about 41 per cent starch. Nutty Brown Flour makes an excellent ingredient to be incorporated with other protein foods. Soya bean flour is not so satisfactory since it has little binding property. Because soya beans do not always produce as palatable a loaf, and also to lend cohesive properties to meatless loaves, one large Los Angeles vegetarian restaurant uses garbanzos which have been previously steamed and ground. While they contain 50 per cent carbohydrates, they are less starchy than are bread crumbs or rice commonly used as fillers.

Soya beans and all low-protein nuts (except peanuts and chestnuts) are compatible with all foods since the type of protein they contain does not require a high gastric acidity for digestion, according to the dietitian of Dr. Hay's Pocono Haven, Crusaders of Compatible Foods. Dr. Horwath has also proved by tests that the enzyme components of the soya bean aid in the digestion of starch. The soya bean has a most prehensil attraction for starches and changes and inverts them, by virtue of its enzymic action, thus markedly aiding digestion.

Egg yolks, being very rich in fat and containing protein in the form of phosphoprotein, are used as neutral foods and combine with all other foods, according to the revised edition of the Hay Official Cook Book, which contains many new recipes using egg yolks in place of whole eggs.

LILLIAN R. CARQUE.

NUT AND BANANA LOAF

½ pound blanched almonds ground fine
½ cup flaked wheat
2 unripe bananas cut up fine
1 cup seeded raisins ground fine
½ cup water

Mix the ingredients thoroughly, put into a pan and bake slowly for about 45 minutes.

NUT CHEESE

1 cup unroasted peanut butter
1 cup whole corn meal ground fine
2½ cups warm water
1 teaspoon savory herbs (marjoram and sage)
1 teaspoon chopped parsley

Steam the corn meal with ½ cup of water in a double boiler for 1 hour. Mix the nut butter with 1 cup of water into the consistency of cream and add all together, including the herbs, to the corn meal, and cook for another ½ hour. When cold, the mixture can be cut into slices like soft cheese.

GRAINUTO No. 1

2 cups oatmeal
1 cup unroasted peanut butter
3 cups warm water
1 teaspoon salt

Steam the oatmeal with 2 cups of water in a double boiler for 1 hour, mix the peanut butter with 1 cup of water to the consistency of cream and stir into the oatmeal and cook for another hour.

GRAINUTO No. 2

2 cups of a preferred protein meal or cereal
1 cup pignolia butter or almond butter
1 cup of warm water (for nut butter)

Steam the meal or cereal with water in a double boiler as recipe indicates, then proceed as directed in the foregoing Grainuto.

THE PREPARATION OF VEGETABLES

All vegetables, except the tubers and starch-bearing roots, should be used as much as possible without cooking. Most green-leaf vegetables and many of the root vegetables are palatable in their raw state. Carrots, turnips, radishes, pumpkins and squashes may be grated or finely ground in a food chopper and used for combination salads. While it is undoubtedly best to eat vegetables which can be enjoyed in their natural state, there are many persons who prefer to have their vegetables cooked or steamed in order to soften the cellulose and to make the cell content more accessible to the digestive juices. Of all methods of cooking, steaming is preferable. The addition of water as used in ordinary cooking toughens the fibres of the vegetable and washes out nearly all of the essential ingredients. By steaming for a short time, the organic salts, the vitamins and the delicious natural flavors are nearly all retained in the food. There are now various waterless cookers and steam boilers on the market which can be used to advantage.

For the economical preparation of vegetables we recommend the *Savory*

Steam Double Boiler. It consists of three parts: a food pan, which fits securely over a water pan, and a cover which fits over both. Holes near the top of the food pan admit steam directly in upon and around the food. (In the ordinary double boiler, the food pan simply extends down into the water pan.) Drain holes in the rim of the food pan permit the steam, which has condensed on the cover, to drop back into the water pan. Thus the food put into the food pan is not immersed in water, which in the ordinary cooker dissolves the organic salts and soaks into the cells of the food. There is no water to drain off, for the food is not boiled in water but softened in steam. The Savory Steam Double Boiler is made of steel covered with porcelain enamel. It can be bought in nearly all large hardware and department stores.

The vegetables which are most satisfactorily prepared in non-aluminum waterless cookers are: asparagus, artichokes, cauliflower, cabbage, celery, egg plant, kale, kohlrabi, okra, onions, pumpkins, salsify, squash, turnips, carrots and potatoes.

The cooking and steaming of vegetables, however, should not be made an every-day practice. We should try to reduce the amount of cooked foods as much as possible. Most roots, such as beets, carrots, radishes, turnips and also squashes and pumpkins can be grated and eaten raw, while some of the stems and green-leaf vegetables—cabbage, celery, chard, lettuce—can be more or less finely ground in a food chopper.

The approximate time necessary for steaming the various vegetables is given in the following table:

Asparagus, whole	20-35 min.	Kale	35-40 min.
Asparagus tips	15-20 min.	Kohlrabi	30-35 min.
Artichokes, small	15-20 hin.	Kohlrabi, sliced	20-25 min.
Artichokes, large	35-40 min.	Mushrooms	15-20 min.
Artichokes, Jerusalem	30-40 min.	Mustard leaves	15-20 min.
Beans, lima, shelled	35-40 min.	Okra, whole	25-30 min.
Beans, string	30-40 min	Okra, sliced	15-20 min.
Beets, sliced	20-25 min.	Onions, large	25-30 min.
Beets, medium	45-50 min.	Onions, small or sliced	20-25 min.
Brocolli	20-25 min.	Oyster plant	35-40 min.
Brussel sprouts	25-30 min.	Oyster plant, sliced	15-20 min.
Cabbage, green and red	35-40 min.	Parsnips, sliced	25-30 min.
Carrots, whole	40-45 min.	Peas, green, shelled	25-30 min.
Carrots, sliced	15-20 min.	Peppers, green	30-35 min.
Cauliflower	25-30 min.	Potatoes	25-30 min.
Celery	20-25 min.	Potatoes, sweet	25-30 min.
Celery roots, sliced	35-40 min.	Pumpkins, peeled	35-40 min.
Chard	15-20 min.	Rhubarb, cut small	10-15 min.
Chayotes, whole	35-40 min.	Rutabagas, sliced	35-40 min.
Chayotes, sliced	15-20 min.	Sorrel	15 min.
Chestnuts	35-40 min.	Spinach	15 min.
Chicory leaves	15-20 min.	Squash, Hubbard	30-35 min.
Corn, green	15-20 min.	Squash, sliced	20-25 min.
Dandelion	15-20 min.	Tomatoes, sliced	10-15 min.
Egg plant, sliced	25-30 min.	Turnips, sliced	35-40 min.
Garlic, cut fine	15-20 min.	Vegetable marrow	20 min.
Horseradish, grated	20-25 min.	Yams	30 min.

Two or three kinds of vegetables whose time of preparation is about the same, may be steamed together. As a seasoning a little chopped parsley, chives or ground nutmeg may be added. One or two tablespoons of thin nut cream (instead of olive oil) will make a palatable and economical dressing, supplying protein and fat which is more or less lacking in vegetables. A few slices of whole wheat bread or rye bread or Rye Krisp should be eaten together with the steamed vegetables (except with starch-bearing kinds) in order to insure enough mastication and insalivation.

For the economical preparation of both whole cereals and legumes, the various kinds of fireless cookers are recommended. A simple and inexpensive fireless cooker can be made in the following manner: Take a wooden box measuring from 12 to 15 inches in each dimension, pack the bottom with crumbled newspaper making a layer of about 1½ to 2 inches thick. Put on top of this layer the well covered pot with the partly cooked vegetables or cereals, and fill the empty space around the pot also with crumbled papers, packing them as tightly as possible. Cover the top with square cushion, stuffed with excelsior, to fit the box. A wooden cover which may be fastened to the box by means of hooks can be easily made. Fireless cooker pots with clamps to securely hold down the cover may be bought in all the larger hardware stores.

SOUPS

Soups take a leading part in the usual menu, but those who have learned to masticate their food thoroughly will find they can easily dispense with them. With the aid of our teeth and salivary glands all solid foods should be reduced to a semi-liquid state before they are swallowed. By forming the soup habit, we interfere with the development of the muscles of mastication and of the gums. While thick vegetable soups eaten with hard crackers or Ry-Crisp may be used ocasionally or given to children or convalescents, meat soups in any form should be discarded altogether. The stimulating effect of the latter is due to the uric acid and other waste poisons or alkaloids which are contained in meat, and are readily dissolved in water. Vegetable soups, if properly made, are rich in organic salts, but care must be taken not to cook the vegetables too long. As an additional seasoning we recommend dehydrated powdered vegetables such as celery, garlic, onions, parsley, dulse (sea lettuce) or kelp.

A number of soups can be made without cooking, simply by heating the ingredients to about 110 degrees Fahrenheit.

Wholesome soup stocks can be made from leafy vegetables, especially the outer leaves of cabbage, lettuce and kale, the tops of celery, green onions, beets and of other roots, spinach, chard, the tough parts of asparagus and cauliflower, etc., which are usually thrown away. The vegetables are best chopped into small pieces by means of a food chopper and then steamed with the addition of a little water in a double boiler, for about 20 minutes or longer if necessary, until the cellulose becomes soft. Then the vegetables should be pressed through a potato ricer to press out the juice and remove the tougher parts of cellulose.

To enrich this vegetable juice with protein, add about one pint of thick nut milk (2 ounces of unroasted nut butter to 14 ounces of water) or use a puree of beans, preferably soybeans, peas or lentils, or soy milk, or its powder sufficiently thinned with water.

Uncooked soups can be made from both vegetables and fruits. A few simple recipes are given herewith. The quantities stated are sufficient for several plates in every instance. One cup or ½ pint of liquid with the ingredients added makes about one plate of soup.

APPLE AND BANANA SOUP

2 apples
2 ripe bananas
1 pint thick nut milk
1 tablespoon honey

Grate the apples, mash the bananas, add honey and nut milk, mix thoroughly all the ingredients and warm in Savory Double Boiler. Flavor with a dash of cinnamon, if desired.

CREAM OF BERRY

1 box berries in season
2 ripe bananas
1 cup (½ pint) nut cream
2 teaspoons honey

Press the berries through the potato ricer, mash the bananas, add nut cream and honey, and mix thoroughly all the ingredients. Serve cold or warm according to season.

CREAM OF GRAPE

1 pound grapes
1 cup orange juice
1 cup nut cream
1 tablespoon honey

Stem the grapes and press the berries through a potato ricer, and mix the grape juice with the other ingredients. Serve cold or warm according to season.

CREAM OF TOMATO

6 medium sized tomatoes
1 cup nut cream
2 tablespoons chopped parsley

Peel and cut the tomatoes into small pieces; then press them through the potato ricer, add the nut cream, parsley or other herbs and mix the ingredients. Add a little water if necessary and serve hot or cold, as desired.

CELERY SOUP

1 head celery
1 small onion
4 cups nut milk (or 1 pint of milk and 1 pint of water)
1 tablespoon whole wheat flour

Cut the celery and onion into small pieces and steam it in the savory double boiler for 15 minutes until tender. To make a smooth soup, the celery may be mashed through a colander or potato ricer. Mix the flour with a little of the nut milk or milk and water. Steam on a low flame for 15 or 20 minutes, thoroughly blending the ingredients. Season with a little salt and nutmeg if desired.

OKRA SOUP

½ pound okra
1 small onion
3 cups nut milk (or 1 cup of water and 2 cups milk)
1 tablespoon whole wheat flour

Chop the okra and onion and steam until soft. Mix the flour with a little of the nut milk or water and proceed like above.

STRING BEAN SOUP

String bean soup may be made in the same way as okra soup, using ½ pound of string beans instead of okra.

POTATO SOUP

1 pound medium sized potatoes
1½ pints water
2 tablespoons unroasted peanut butter
6 stalks of celery, cut fine
½ cup chopped parsley
½ teaspoon salt, if desired

Wash and steam the potatoes together with celery in the Savory Double Boiler for 30 minutes. Take out the potatoes, remove skins and mash through the ricer. Dissolve the nut butter in ½ pint water and put all the ingredients back into the savory, steam for about 20 minutes and serve with a dash of mace or nutmeg.

LIMA BEAN SOUP

1 cup lima beans
4 cups water
1 onion
1 turnip
1 carrot
2 tablespoons nut cream
½ teaspoon salt (if desired)

Wash the beans and soak them in cold water overnight. In the morning put them in the food pan of a Double Boiler, add the vegetables, ground fine by means of a food chopper, and steam for at least two hours, or until they are tender enough to rub through a sieve or colander. Then put the beans back into the kettle with the broth in which they were cooked. Add the nut cream and steam for a few minutes more.

LIMA BEAN SOUP POWDER

Soak one pound beans overnight. Remove the skins, which the soaking has loosened, by pressing the beans between the fingers. Steam slowly for about two hours, in as little water as possible, adding one tablespoon of vegetable cooking fat or nut butter. When thoroughly cooked they will fall apart and become pasty or flaky. Now press the mass through as fine a sieve as possible and dry in open dish in oven (door open), or in the sun. When thoroughly dry and powdery sift again. The result will be a fine flour. The finer the better. If necessary, use a rolling pin for reducing the paste. A fine well-dried bean flour will keep successfully in a hermetically sealed container, if stored in a cool place.

INSTANTANEOUS BEAN SOUP

2 tablespoons lima bean flour
1 cup boiling hot water or nut milk
1 tablespoon finely chopped parsley

Mix the flour thoroughly with the water or nut milk, add the parsley and heat for a few minutes, stirring well.

PEA SOUP

1 cup dried split peas
1 quart cold water
1 medium sized onion, minced
1½ cups celery, cut fine
1 tablespoon chopped parsley
½ cup nut cream
½ teaspoon salt or salt substitute (if desired)

Soak the peas in water over night and cook with the vegetables in the morning, using double boiler. When tender, add the nut cream and salt if desired and serve.

LENTIL SOUP

1 cup lentils
4 cups water (1 quart)
2 tablespoons nut cream
1 medium onion, chopped fine
4 stalks of celery, chopped fine
1 teaspoon lemon juice

Soak the lentils over night in the water, using the same water for cooking. Simmer slowly for about 2 hours, or until the lentils are soft, taking off any scum that rises. Add the vegetables and stew for another hour. Rub through a colander, if desired. Add the lemon juice and nut cream and serve.

BEAN SOUP

1 cup white navy beans
4 cups water
½ cup chopped parsley
1 tablespoon nut cream
1 teaspoon lemon juice

Soak the beans over night in 2 cups of water. Add the rest of the water in the morning and boil until soft. Run through a colander, if desired; add parsley and nut cream; let boil again and serve. If boiled beans are used only half the amount of water is required.

ASPARAGUS SOUP

12 asparagus, cleaned and cut into pieces
1 bunch of spinach, washed and chopped
2 potatoes, peeled and sliced
½ cup nut cream
3 cups water
1 pinch salt, if desired

Put all the ingredients, except the nut cream, into the Savory Double Boiler and boil for about 30 minutes. Pass through a colander; add the nut cream; season and serve.

BARLEY SOUP

1 cup whole barley
4 cups water
1 chopped onion
½ cup chopped celery
1 tablespoon chopped parsley
2 cups of peanut milk

Cook the barley in the 4 cups of water for about 3 hours until soft. The Waterless Cooker is best adapted for this purpose. Then add the vegetables and nut milk and let boil for another 20 minutes. Add ½ teaspoon salt, if desired. For small children and convalescents this soup should be passed through a colander.

CAULIFLOWER SOUP

1 cauliflower, cleaned, cut in flowerettes
2 onions, chopped fine
1 tablespoon chopped parsley
4 cups nut milk
½ teaspoon salt

Steam cauliflower and onions until tender; add the nut milk and parsley; steam for another 5 minutes and serve. Instead of the onions ½ bunch of celery cut fine may be used.

ONION AND POTATO SOUP

3 medium sized onions, peeled and grated
2 potatoes, peeled and grated
2 tablespoons chopped parsley
1 quart peanut milk

Put all ingredients in the Savory Double Boiler and steam for 15 to 20 minutes.

ONION, CELERY AND TOMATO SOUP

4 onions chopped fine
1 cup celery chopped fine
3 tomatoes sliced or 1 small can tomatoes
3 cups nut milk

Put all ingredients in the Savory Double Boiler and steam for 15 minutes.

SAUCES (Uncooked and Cooked)

CRANBERRY SAUCE

2 cups cranberries
2 ripe bananas mashed
1 tablespoon nut cream
1 tablespoon honey

Wash the cranberries and put through a food chopper and mix thoroughly with the other ingredients. Let stand for an hour before serving. This sauce may be used for nut loaves and puddings.

TOMATO SAUCE

1 cup strained tomato juice
1 cup nut cream

Mix together and heat for 10 minutes in a double boiler to blend thoroughly the ingredients. Use for nut loaves or salads.

APPLE SAUCE

2 juicy tart apples
½ cup nut cream
1 tablespoon honey

Peel and grate the apples and mix with the nut cream and honey. This makes a nice sauce for cold pudding and fruit salads. Baked apples may also be used for this recipe.

BANANA SAUCE

2 large ripe bananas
1 cup nut cream
1 tablespoon honey

Peel and mash the bananas and thoroughly mix together with the nut cream and honey. This makes a good sauce for cooked cereals such as wheat or rice, also for fresh berries.

PUDDINGS

BANANA AND APPLE PUDDING

2 medium size apples, grated
4 tablespoons nut meal (almond or pine nut)
2 ripe bananas
2 teaspoon grated cocoanut
1 teaspoon finely grated orange peel

Mix the grated apples and nut meal. Add 1½ bananas cut in small pieces, mix again and put in mould to give it shape. Turn the pudding out in a plate and sprinkle with the grated cocoanut and orange peel. Decorate with thin slices of the other half banana. Let stand at least 15 minutes before serving.

CARROT PUDDING No. 1

3 medium sized carrots (¾ pound) grated
2 cups bread crumbs, ground fine
1 cup seedless raisins
1 tablespoon honey
1 cup nut milk
1 dash nutmeg

Mix the ingredients thoroughly and steam in a double boiler for ½ hour. Instead of the bread crumbs 2 cups of flaked wheat or boiled rice may be used.

CARROT PUDDING No. 2

2½ cups grated raw carrots
1 cup grated raw potatoes
2 stalks celery cut fine
1 medium sized onion chopped fine
1 tablespoon chopped parsley
2 eggs or 1 cup nut cream

Mix ingredients after beating eggs slightly, turn into baking dish, sprinkle with bread crumbs and parsley. Bake for 45 minutes or steam in a waterless cooker for ½ hour.

FRUIT PUDDING

2½ cups flaked whole wheat (10 ounces)
1 cup nut milk
½ cup chopped nuts or nut meal
½ cup chopped figs
½ cup chopped pitted dates
½ cup seedless raisins

Moisten the wheat with the nut milk and then mix all ingredients well and steam in a double boiler for 40 minutes. Serve with banana dressing or cranberry sauce.

WHOLE WHEAT CURRANT PUDDING

2 cups toasted whole wheat bread crumbs
1 cup currants
1 cup nut milk
1 dash cinnamon

Mix well, moisten with nut milk and steam in a double boiler for ½ hour. Serve with nut cream. Instead of bread crumbs 2½ cups of flaked whole wheat may be used.

THE PREPARATION OF CEREALS

Cereals and legumes are among the leading staple foods of the world because of their availability, also because they are easily stored and transported and are relatively cheap. Cereals and legumes are usually not eaten in their natural state, although people with perfect teeth and plenty of time for mastication may occasionally use the natural whole grains. Cereals are by no means essential in our nutrition and they may be replaced to a large extent by dried fruits and nuts. But until fruit and nut culture has sufficiently advanced, cereals will constitute a large part of man's diet.

Only such cereal foods should be used as are made from the entire grain. It is folly to eat largely of white flour products and then use bran separately as a laxative. Those persons who are not able to secure whole grain flours freshly ground should by all means buy a small hand mill and make their own flours. We especially recommend "The Quaker City Mill," which can be attached to a table. The mill is adapted for fine or coarse grinding and can also be used for making flour from beans, peas, lentils, etc. Legumes are more completely assimilated when ground fine. The milling process pulverizes the fibrous parts and cellulose which are difficult to digest for many people. Most of the difficulties, however, are due to the fact that legumes are eaten in wrong combinations and in too large proportions. If no more than a cupful is taken at a time and combined with a vegetable salad, they are well digested and assimilated.

GERMINATED CEREALS

Cereals, especially wheat, may be used in their natural state if they are soaked in water for about 24 hours. This will start germination and change part of the starch into maltose. This softened wheat may be run through a food chopper together with a few raisins.

If fresh vegetables or fruit are not available, an antiscorbutic food can be prepared by moistening any kind of whole cereals or legumes and allowing them to germinate or sprout. The making of bean sprouts is described elsewhere under the heading of "soybeans."

BOILED WHOLE WHEAT

Boiled whole wheat is one of the simplest ways of preparing the cereal, as it does away with the milling and baking process. Boiling makes the whole grain more digestible and palatable, while preserving its nutritive value as much as possible. A waterless cooker is admirably adapted for this purpose as it develops a slight steam pressure and thereby shortens the time necessary for boiling wheat in the ordinary cooking utensil. The wheat grain should be carefully washed in several waters until all the dust is removed, then add to every pound of wheat 1 quart of water and let it stand for 20 to 24 hours. By this time nearly all the water will be absorbed; if necessary add another cup of water. Let it simmer in the waterless cooker for about 3 hours. Serve with nut cream and vegetable salad. No more than one cup of boiled wheat, well masticated, should be eaten as a part of a meal.

FLAKED CEREALS, ETC.

Rolled or flaked and shredded grains are now made by many mills and factories and sold as breakfast foods in various forms. To make the flaked cereals, the husked and scoured grain is steamed for a short time in big revolving drums in order to soften it. While still wet it is run between rapidly revolving steel rollers and pressed into thin flakes. After drying and sterilizing the flakes the product is ready for the market. As the flaked cereals are only partially cooked they are supposed to be re-cooked before serving, although some people eat them without further preparation. Some recipes using flaked cereals are given in the following pages. The shredded products are made with special machinery which tears the steam cooker kernels into shreds and deposits them in layers or bundles, in which form they are baked.

In some of the widely advertised breakfast foods which are supposed to be malted or predigested, only a small percentage of starch has been converted into dextrin during the manufacturing process. The change from the unsoluble starch into dextrin is produced by an enzyme, *diastase,* whose action is arrested by the heating process. Of the five cereals most commonly used for breakfast foods oats and wheat contain perhaps the largest quantities of important nutrients, with a fairly low proportion of crude fiber. Rice is low in protein but remarkably free from crude fiber. Microscopic examination of the starches from the common cereals, and from potatoes show that the granules of the rice starch are very much smaller than are those of other cereals, and for that reason they are more easily attacked by the digestive ferments of the human body, because of the greater sur-area exposed. Recently a new rice product, "Puffed Rice," has been put on the market, supposedly made from the entire grain. Corn is also used in considerable quantities for the manufacture of breakfast foods, but is slightly less digestible than are the other cereals. Barley is seldom used in the flaked form; it is generally served as pearl barley, which is a demineralized product the same as is polished rice. Only the whole barley flour should be used.

Some of the flaked cereals, like oats, have been cooked at a slow heat for several hours. In order to prevent overheating during the cooking, they are periodically cooled by a special ventilating system. In these preparations a considerable quantity of starch has been dextrinized and they may, therefore, be prepared for the table in but a few minutes.

BUCKWHEAT AND MILLET

Buckwheat is raised to a rather small extent in the eastern parts of the United States and northwest Europe. It is generally placed on the market as buckwheat flour (so called) for making the well known buckwheat cakes. There is probably no bread or cake material that is subjected to more extensive adulteration than is buckwheat flour. Mixtures of rye flour, wheat flour, corn flour, with a little salt and a leavening agent, but containing very little buckwheat, are generally sold as buckwheat flour.

Millet is mostly grown for forage in the United States but in eastern Russia, China and India it is a staple food for man. In India, the consumption of millet is larger than that of wheat. Of course, only the unpolished millet should be used. It is lower in protein content than are the other cereals, except rice, but contains an appreciable amount of fat, potash, magnesia and iron. It is usually cooked whole, like rice.

BREAD MAKING

Bread is probably the largest single item in the diet of a great majority of people in Europe and America. Statistics show that wheat flour and other wheat products supply 20 per cent of the total food materials used by the average American family, but in many districts in Europe, northern Africa and western Asia bread in various forms comprises a much larger part of the daily dietary. Both leavened and unleavened bread has been used since the dawn of history. Fermentation is a chemical process caused by the growth of a microscopical plant, the yeast cell in a liquid or semi-liquid substance, containing sugar originally present or produced from starch by diastase or enzymic action. In feeding, the yeast cell breaks up the sugar into alcohol and carbonic acid gas. It is this gas which forces its way through the tenacious part of the gluten and lightens the dough. The yeast grows only in the presence of moisture and suitable nutritive material, and multiplies quickly at a temperature of from 70 to 95 degrees Fahrenheit. In the process of baking the growth of the yeast is arrested and as the temperature passes over 200 degrees Fahrenheit the yeast plant is destroyed. So called wild yeast is present in the atmosphere and most yeasts used in ancient times have been cultivated from it. A great deal of yeast is now taken from brewers' and distillers' vats in which malt extract has been fermenting. The commonly used compressed yeast is usually produced from distillers' wort, washed in cold water, by passing it through wire sieves or by precipitation in the liquid. It is then pressed, cut in cakes, and done up in tinfoil.

Unleavened breads are those made light by thoroughly kneading the dough without the use of yeast, baking powder or soda. If properly made, they are the most wholesome of all breads for they retain the natural sweetness of the grain, which is more or less lost in the process of fermentation that takes place in the leavened bread.

In bread making like in the preparation of all foods, soft or distilled water is preferable to hard water. For the success of any of the following recipes it is essential to have genuine whole wheat flour to make a pasty dough.

The proper proportions for making bread are one quart of liquids to three pounds of flour. With some kinds of flour a little more than three pounds are required, but the excess will never be more than ½ pound. All the liquids should be poured into the pan first. Then put in the flour and other ingredients.

When making yeast, cover and set the pan away in a warm room, so the dough will rise. After rising knead and put into baking pans. A convenient size of the pan is as follows: 8 inches long 3½ inches wide and 3 inches high.

Most all modern baking ovens are now equipped with a thermometer to control the temperature during the baking process. When the bread dough is ready to be baked, it should be put in a fairly hot oven of about 400 degrees Fahrenheit to allow it to form a crust and stop rising. After the first 15 or 20 minutes the temperature of the oven should be decreased about 20 degrees until the bread is baked. Loaves of bread of ordinary size made with yeast require from 50 to 60 minutes of baking. They should start to brown after the first 20 minutes. For unleavened breads a temperature of about 360 degrees Fahrenheit will be sufficient, but for that reason they will require a little longer for baking.

In the following recipes the use of table salt is made optional. Those who have been living on natural foods for some time can easily dispense with coarse salt. Instead of salt dehydrated powdered vegetables such as celery, parsley, dulse (sea lettuce) or kelp may be used.

The use of yeast in bread-making is not injurious if all the ingedients are fresh and good, including the yeast. Those who object to yeast germs should know that they are destroyed during the baking process, if it is done well. Yeast bread, however, should never be eaten hot, but at least one or two days old, preferably toasted.

*Baking powders are more or less objectionable. There are three kinds; the cream of tartar type, the phosphate powders, and the alum powders. The effect of baking powders results from the formation of carbonic acid gas, which penetrates the loaf, forms small cavities through the expansion of gluten and makes the bread light. All baking powders leave a mineral residue in the bread and for this reason they are relatively less wholesome than are the products made with yeast. The alum powders are the least desirable as they leave a deposit of hydrate of aluminum and sulphate of soda. Two teaspoons of tartrate powder leave in a loaf made from a quart of flour about 165 grains (over 1/3 ounce) of Rochelle salts, while the phosphate powders leave a still larger amount of phosphate of lime and phosphate of soda.

**Raw crystallized cane sugar and honey are recommended in all recipes where sweetening is required. Raw sugar is made from the purified but unrefined juice of sugar cane by condensing the juice in large vacuum pans. Raw sugar was until recently a regular commercial product, and could be obtained in the larger cities of the United States. It is preferable to refined sugar, as it still contains some of the mineral salts which are entirely removed by the refining process.

Honey has been used as a food from the earliest times, and constitutes, besides maple syrup, one of the principal sweetening materials up to about fifty years ago when sugar became a commercial product. Honey contains about 75 per cent of carbohydrates made up of equal parts of dextrose (grape sugar) and levulose (fruit sugar); about 2 per cent sucrose (cane sugar), never over 8 per cent; 18 per cent water and 0.23 per cent mineral matter. In addition it contains a small amount of formic acid, protein, aromatic bodies, enzymes, pigments, acids, dextrins and gums.

---

*Cream of Tartar base baking powders such as Royal, a derivative of grapes, are considered less harmful than are those of the alum (aluminum) type. A new baking powder, sold under the name of Stur-Dee Tartaric Baking Powder, is an absolutely pure product and leaves an alkaline ash in the body, according to the dietitian of Dr. Hay's Pocono Haven who uses and recommends it. Yeast is considered less objectionable as a leavening agent than is baking powder; however, each has its place to produce the desired results.

Strange as it may seem ammonia is the finest of all leaveners, but should not be used by those who do not understand its strength, according to Nutritionist-Baker, Dr. Guy E. Roush of Glendale, California, whose experience and study covers a period of thirty years. The formation of a perfect amount of carbon dioxide gas, which when scientifically handled, is driven off, leaving the finished product sweet, fragrant and practically free from residue, states Dr. Roush.

LILLIAN R. CARQUE.

**Legal authorities state that under regulations of the Pure Food, Drug and Cosmetic Act, now effective, raw sugar does not comply with the requirements as to food unless it is further freed of impurities; and that any person delivering it will be subject to severe penalties. It is pointed out that raw sugar was never manufactured to be used as a food in that form, but was solely intended for transportation from plantations to the refineries. An analysis of raw sugar shows foreign matter which might be sufficient evidence of adulteration under present laws. A yellow crystal sugar which is processed to remove the non-essential foreign matter from raw sugar has been made available. This superior product contains all the beneficial mineral salts occurring in the best grades of raw sugar—in a quantity FIVE TIMES greater—and meets every requirement of the Federal Pure Food and Drug Act. Yellow Crystal Sugar also has a taste far more pleasant than that of raw sugar.

LILLIAN R. CARQUE.

Another feature of the recipes is that nut products are used instead of the usual extracted animal and vegetable fats. As nuts are rich in both fat and protein, they also can take the place largely of dairy products, especially eggs. As it has been shown in Chapter XIV the use of nuts and nut products should be increased for economic as well as hygienic reasons. During the past 25 years the lowly peanut has steadily grown in popularity as a food for man. There is no reason why its use should not further increase, if eaten judiciously. Peanuts are rich in protein and fat and when hygienically prepared may replace to a large extent meat and dairy products. One pound of unroasted nut butter is equal in nutritive value to that contained in 3 dozen eggs, or 1 level tablespoonful nut butter to 2 eggs. Where no special mention is made, any kind of nut may be used in the following recipes.

WHOLE WHEAT BREAD No. 1

3½ cups whole wheat flour (about 1 pound)
1½ cups milk or nut milk
(Nut milk: 2 tablespoons unroasted nut butter thoroughly mixed with 1½ cups warm water)
2 tablespoons raw sugar or honey
½ cake yeast
½ teaspoon salt (if desired)

Slightly heat the milk together with the honey and salt. When lukewarm, add the yeast, first mixing it with a little milk. Add the flour. Knead well and let it double its volume. Again knead it thoroughly, put into oiled pans, leaving sufficient space to rise. It should then be baked in a hot oven for about 50 minutes.

WHOLE WHEAT CRACKERS

May be made from the same kind of dough by rolling it out about one-fifth of an inch thick. Cut into any shape desired and bake in well oiled pans for 10 to 15 minutes.

WHOLE WHEAT BREAD No. 2 (3 Loaves)

5 cups hard wheat flour
1¾ cups lukewarm water (80°F.)
1 tablespoon honey
1 tablespoon nut butter dressing
½ cake yeast
½ teaspoon salt

Dissolve yeast in the ¾ cup of water and add the honey to the liquid. Put 4½ cups of flour in a bowl and pour in the dissolved yeast, washing out the cup with the balance or 1 cup of water, add nut cream and stir thoroughly for a few minutes. Cover and set in warm place to raise for 1½ hours and work in the ½ cup of flour reserved. Put in oiled pans and place in a warm place to raise a little more. Bake in a moderately hot oven (360°F.) for 45 minutes.

WHOLE WHEAT BREAD No. 3 (6 Loaves)

1 large boiled potato
3 pints water (including the potato water)
2 tablespoons nut butter
2 tablespoons honey or raw sugar
1 cake yeast
4 pounds whole wheat flour, or enough to make a stiff dough
1 teaspoon salt if desired

Dissolve the yeast in a little tepid water. Cut the potato into small pieces and put through a ricer, add the nut butter and honey with the water in which the potato was boiled. Then gradually add the balance of the water, to make up three pints, the yeast and enough of the whole wheat flour to make a firm batter. Mix thoroughly and put in a warm place until it rises to nearly double its original bulk, then work a little more flour and put into oiled pans, making them about half full and let them stand until the sponge has risen to the rim. Brush the top of the loaves with a little oil, put the pans in a hot oven and bake for 45 minutes to 1 hour. Remove the loaves from the pans, and when thoroughly cooled store away.

WHOLE WHEAT BREAD STICKS

Take bits of the whole wheat dough after it is first kneaded, roll with the fingers on the breadboard into thin sticks, about the size of a lead pencil, and bake in an oiled pan in a hot oven for 15 or 20 minutes. This is one of the best forms of bread, especially used with soups and salads.

WHOLE WHEAT RAISIN BREAD

7 cups (2 pounds) whole wheat flour
2 cups seedless raisins (washed and cleaned)
1 tablespoon honey
2 tablespoons oil
2½ cups water or nut milk
1 yeast cake
1 teaspoon salt (if desired)

Dissolve the yeast cake in ½ cup of warm water, add salt, honey, oil and raisins. Put into a pan, add the flour and balance of water. Knead well for 10 minutes and keep in a warm place for several hours. Knead again and put the dough into well-oiled pans. Let it rise in the pan about an hour, then bake for 45 minutes. Brush the loaves with oil as directed in the preceding recipes.

WHOLE CORN BREAD AND MUFFINS

(2 loaves)

5 cups whole corn meal
1 cup whole wheat flour
2 tablespoons olive oil
1 tablespoon honey
2 cups warm water or nut milk
½ yeast cake

Dissolve the yeast cake in 1 cup of water, add the honey and oil. Put into a pan, add the meal, flour and balance of water or nut milk and proceed like above. The same dough can be used for corn muffins, which require only about 20 minutes for baking.

UNFERMENTED WHOLE WHEAT BREAD

(2 or 3 loaves)

½ cup olive oil
1¼ cups water
7 cups (2 pounds) whole wheat flour or sufficient to make a stiff dough
1 level teaspoonful salt (if desired)

Beat the oil steadily, adding the water a little at a time until the emulsion is formed resembling the beaten whites of eggs. When all the water has been added, sprinkle the flour very quickly over the entire emulsion so as to hold all the air confined in the mixture. Make a stiff dough; knead thoroughly until smooth and elastic. Let the dough stand over night, or at least a few hours, and then knead again before forming into loaves. Bake in a moderately hot oven 1 to 1½ hours.

UNLEAVENED FRUIT BREAD

2 cups water
1 cup cracked wheat
1 cup seedless raisins
½ cup pitted dates chopped fine
½ cup figs chopped fine
1 cup nut cream
½ cup honey

Soak the wheat in water over night, add the other ingredients in the morning and thoroughly mix them together. Steam in the Savory Double Boiler for about 2 hours, then shape into loaves of convenient size and bake in a moderately hot oven following day.

UNLEAVENED WHOLE WHEAT BISCUIT

4 cups whole wheat flakes
¼ cup honey
½ cup nut butter dressing
3 eggs

Beat whites and yolks of eggs separately, thoroughly mix together the yolks, nut butter and honey. Then mix in white of the eggs and finally the wheat flakes. Drop a spoonful at a time on oiled pans and bake for 15 minutes or until light brown.

UNLEAVENED WHOLE WHEAT FRUIT CRACKERS

1 pound whole wheat flour
½ cup of almond butter
¾ cup water
½ cup seedless raisins, ground figs or dates

Dissolve the almond butter by adding a little water at a time. Mix it well until all the water is used. Add the salt and all the flour that can be kneaded in. Work the dough from 10 to 15 minutes; roll out until ⅛ of an inch thick and cut into equal parts. Spread one part with seeded raisins or ground figs or dates; then place the other piece of dough upon the fruit. Press together with a rolling-pin and perforate partly through with a fork at frequent intervals. Cut into any desired shape and bake in a moderately hot oven until of a light brown color.

WHOLE WHEAT GEMS No. 1

1 cup of nut meal
2 cups cold water
3 cups whole wheat flour or sufficient to make a batter
A pinch of salt

Thoroughly mix the ingredients and beat the batter for 10 minutes; then put into hot gem irons and bake for about 45 minutes.

WHOLE WHEAT GEMS No. 2

2 cups nut milk or 2 pints sour milk
3 cups whole wheat flour or enough to make a batter
1 egg
A pinch of salt

Thoroughly mix the nut milk, the yolk of the egg and the salt. Then add the flour, putting only a little in at a time to retain as much air as possible in the mixture. Then mix in the well-beaten white of the egg. Put into gem irons, which have been heated and oiled, and bake for about 45 minutes. When baking with gas, put the gems on the top grate of the oven and use one burner only at first.

WHOLE WHEAT PEANUT GEMS

1½ cups cold water
3½ cups or enough whole wheat flour to make a batter that will pour readily
2 eggs
½ cup unroasted peanut butter
A pinch of salt

Mix the peanut butter and salt with the water in a round-bottom dish; add the yolk of the eggs; then beat the whites of the eggs until they are stiff and set aside until the dough is ready. Beat the nut milk (resulting from the mixture of peanut butter, water and yolks), with an egg-beater until frothy. Add the flour a little at a time, beating continuously with a spoon until the mixture is of the desired consistency. Then add, without further beating, the white of the eggs. Pour into warm and well-oiled gem irons and bake for about 45 minutes.

HONEY COCONUT MACAROONS

½ cup coconut oil or ½ cup nut cream
½ cup (½ lb.) honey
1 cup hot water
2 cups (½ lb.) shredded coconut
2 cups (¾ lb.) whole wheat flour

Mix thoroughly the oil, honey and hot water and then stir in the shredded coconut and flour. Put in convenient shapes on a well-oiled pan and bake in a moderately hot oven for ½ hour. This should make about 3 dozen macaroons.

PLAIN WHOLE WHEAT SCONES

1¼ lbs. whole wheat flour
3 tablespoons butter or any pure vegetable shortening
1½ cups water

Rub the shortening into the flour, wet with enough water to make a firm dough, roll out and cut in biscuit form about ½ inch thick. Bake in hot oven for 10 minutes, brush scones with oil and then finish in a moderately hot oven in about ¾ hour.

SWEET WHOLE WHEAT RAISIN SCONES

1½ pounds whole wheat flour
1 cup vegetable oil or 8 ounces shortening
1 cup honey (melted)
¾ lb. seedless raisins (washed)
2 cups water or enough to form a stiff dough

Rub the shortening into the flour, add the honey, water and raisins. Knead very well roll out and bake as above. As a shortening pure coconut fat may be used.

ALMOND ROCKS

1 lb. whole wheat flour
½ cup vegetable oil or 4 ounces shortening
6 ounces honey (melted)
2 ounces chopped unblanched almonds
1¼ cups water

Mix honey and shortening thoroughly with the flour, add almonds and enough water to form a stiff dough. Form into irregular rocks with a spoon and put on a greased pan. Bake in moderately hot oven 20 minutes for small rocks, or longer according to size.

COCONUT ROCKS

¾ pound whole wheat flour
½ pound grated coconut
½ cup vegetable oil or 4 ounces shortening
½ pound honey
1 cup (small) hot water

Melt the fat and honey in the hot water, stir in flour and cocoanut, beat well and bake in small rocks for ½ hour in a moderately hot oven.

WHOLE WHEAT FRUIT COOKIES

¾ pound whole wheat flour
½ cup vegetable oil or 4 ounces shortening
½ cup honey
2 ounces chopped nuts
½ pound chopped figs, pitted dates and seedless raisins mixed
1 cup hot water

Melt shortening and honey with hot water, stir in flour, nuts, fruit and more hot water if necessary, to form a soft dough. Bake in rock form in a moderately hot oven for about 45 minutes.

BREAD NUTS

3 cups whole wheat flour
1½ cups nut butter dressing

Mix flour and nut cream thoroughly and knead for about 20 minutes; roll out an inch thick and cut with very small round cutter. Bake in quick oven 10 minutes and follow with moderate heat for about 20 minutes.

WHOLE WHEAT PASTRY FOR PIES

¾ pound whole wheat flour
4 tablespoons vegetable oil or unsalted vegetable fat
1 small cup water

Rub the shortening into the flour and mix with enough water to make a nice soft dough. Knead for about 15 minutes, bake in a quick oven for a few minutes and finish with moderate heat.

UNFIRED FRUIT CAKE

½ cup ground whole wheat crumbs
1 cup pitted dates, finely minced
½ cup dried figs, finely minced
½ cup nut meal (no peanuts)
1 large juicy apple, grated
½ teaspoon cinnamon or nutmeg

Mix ingredients thoroughly by running them through a food chopper, add a little water if necessary to make a thick paste. Press into a bowl and cover till the following day.

WHOLE WHEAT FILBERT BISCUITS

½ pound shelled filberts
3 eggs
2½ cups water
3 cups whole wheat flour
Salt (if desired)

Grind filberts into a nut meal. Beat eggs thoroughly; add the water and beat in the whole wheat flour. Then put in filbert meal and bake in hot gem irons in a quick oven.

WHOLE WHEAT ALMOND ROLLS

1 cup whole wheat flour
½ cup almond meal
½ cup water (enough to make stiff dough)

Knead all ingredients together for 10 minutes; form into rolls of not more than 1 inch thick and about 2 inches long. Bake in well-oiled tins in a moderately hot oven for nearly an hour.

WHOLE WHEAT PEANUT ROLLS

2 cups peanut butter dressing
Enough flour to make a very stiff dough
A pinch salt

Knead all ingredients together for at least 10 minutes; form into rolls and bake as above.

WHOLE RICE PEANUT ROLLS

2 cups boiled whole rice
2/3 cup nut meal
1/3 cup whole wheat flour
1 egg beaten
Salt (if desired)

After the rice has sufficiently cooled add the nut meal, beaten egg, and then the whole wheat flour. Knead the mixture thoroughly until smooth and firm. Form into rolls about ¾ of an inch thick and 3 inches long; bake in well-oiled pans in a moderately hot oven.

STEAMED BROWN BREAD

1 cup unrefined sugar
2 cups thin nut butter dressing
1 cup whole wheat flour
2 cups whole corn meal

Heat the nut cream slightly in the Savory Double Boiler. Then add the corn meal and unrefined sugar, and finally mix in the whole wheat flour. Steam for several hours; then put into cans and place in moderately hot oven to brown for a little while.

CORN RELISH

1 cup whole corn meal
2½ cups boiling water
1 cup nut cream
1 tablespoon parsley, chopped fine
¼ cup grated cheese

Stir the corn meal in the boiling water and cook in a double boiler for ½ hour. Then add nut cream, parsley, and cheese and let the mixture come to a boil again. Put into a shallow pan to cool, cut into squares, sprinkle a little grated cheese on top and bake in a moderate oven for a few minutes or long enough to melt the cheese.

CORN AND POTATO MUFFINS

1 cup mashed potatoes
1 cup whole corn meal
1 cup milk or nut milk
1 egg well beaten

Moisten the potato with the milk, stir in the corn until the batter is just thick enough to drop easily from the spoon; add the whipped egg and beat hard. Drop into hot, oiled gem pans and bake in an oven 20 to 30 minutes.

POTATO CAKES

4 cups mashed potatoes
½ cup whole wheat flour
1 cup nut butter dressing

Thoroughly mix all ingredients, then form into little flat cakes, half an inch thick and 2 inches in diameter and bake in an oiled gem pan for 20 minutes until they have light brown color.

OATMEAL CRACKERS

1 pound oatmeal
2 cups water
1 cup nut meal
2 tablespoons honey or raw sugar
1 teapsoon salt

Mix together water, nut meal, and honey and knead in the oatmeal. Work the dough thoroughly for 10 minutes and roll out until it is about ⅜ in. thick. Cut into pieces 1 inch wide and 2 inches long. Bake until they are dry all through, but not too brown.

SCOTCH OAT CAKES

2 cups fine oatmeal or ground rolled oats
1 to 1½ cups warm nut milk to make a soft batter

Mix well together, making the dough as smooth as possible, and roll out to the thickness of about ⅛ inch. Make one or two round cakes, and cut into quarters. Put in a shallow oiled pan and bake in a hot oven for 20 minutes.

OATMEAL BANNOCKS

2 cups fine oatmeal
1 cup hot nut milk or enough to make a thick batter

Mix well together and let the mixture stand for 20 minutes, first flouring the board and rolling pin with wheat flour. Cut into small cakes and bake in a moderate oven 15 minutes, or till they are dry and hard, but only slightly browned. If put into a closed jar they will keep for several weeks.

OATMEAL AND COCONUT CRACKELS

2 cups fine oatmeal
½ cup dessicated grated coconut
3 tablespoons honey or raw sugar
1 cup hot nut milk

Dissolve the honey in the hot water and mix all ingredients thoroughly together; turn out the dough on a well-floured rolling board and roll out to ¼ inch in thickness and proceed as directed above. To make the baked crackels crispy let them stand a day or two in an uncovered dish. A very palatable pie crust can be made from this dough, if a little more hot water is added.

SWEET POTATO BREAD

1½ cups finely mashed sweet boiled potatoes
2½ cups whole wheat flour
2 tablespoons nut cream
2 tablespoons warm water
½ yeast cake
½ teaspoon salt

Dissolve yeast in the warm water; add salt, nut cream, potatoes and enough flour to make a smooth sponge; cover and set in a warm place to rise. When light add the remainder of the flour or whatever is needed to make a smooth, elastic dough. Cover and let rise until light; mould into one or two loaves, rolls, or gems and bake in moderate oven. The loaves will require 35 to 40 minutes, the rolls and gems about 20 minutes until done.

BARLEY BREAD

2 cups whole barley flour
1 cup whole wheat flour
2 tablespoons nut cream
1 tablespoon honey
½ yeast cake
1 cup warm water
½ teaspoon salt

Make a sponge by dissolving the yeast in the warm water, stirring into this the wheat flour to make a soft dough. Set in a warm place to rise and add nut cream, honey, salt and the barley flour. Knead for 10 minutes and let rise again. Divide into 2 loaves and bake in well-oiled pans 35 to 40 minutes. This bread bakes more quickly than does other bread.

WHOLE RYE BREAD

The grain of rye is much darker in color than that of wheat, but otherwise it is similar in appearance. Whole rye flour contains more protein than does wheat flour; it is also richer in iron and fluorine. In the northeastern parts of Europe rye has practically replaced wheat as a bread-making cereal, for it is more easily cultivated than is wheat. The following is an excellent recipe for rye bread:

5 cups whole rye flour
1½ cups whole wheat flour
2 tablespoons olive oil or nut butter
2 tablespoons honey or unrefined sugar
½ cup nut milk
2½ cups warm water
1 yeast cake
1 teaspoon salt

Place the olive oil or unroasted nut butter together with the honey and salt in a large pan and pour in the 2½ cups of hot water. When lukewarm add the yeast cake, dissolved in the warm milk, together with the whole rye flour. Knead thoroughly for about 10 minutes. Cover the mixture and let rise for 3 hours in a room of about 70 degrees Fahrenheit. Add 1½ cups of whole wheat flour or sufficient to make a rather stiff dough; knead thoroughly for about 15 minutes. Then shape into 3 or 4 loaves; place in oiled pans and let rise about 30 minutes. Bake in a moderately hot oven about 1 hour.

Unleavened rye breads, made according to the Swedish process from the entire rye grain, are most palatable and wholesome. They are excellent for children, especially when placed in a moderately hot oven for a few minutes, for they require thorough mastication and contain valuable food elements. They can be bought in all the larger cities of the United States.

NATURAL WHOLE RICE

Whole rice, also called *brown rice,* contains the bran, cuticle and germ of the cereal. In milling nothing has been removed but the husk and dirt. Rice is made white or pearly by machine polishing and by a coating of glucose, etc. This is done to improve its appearance, but the peeling and polishing removes the germ and the layers immediately around it, leaving the kernel deficient in vitamins and organic salts. To prepare whole rice take 1 cup of rice to 3 cups of water. Bring to boil on a slow fire for 5 minutes, and then let simmer for 45 minutes. When using a fireless cooker, boil for 10 minutes and then leave in the cooker for 4 hours or longer, if desired. When using the Savory Steam Double Boiler, take only 2½ cups of water and let the rice boil in the food pan for 5 minutes. Then place the food pan in the water pan and steam cook for 1 hour without stirring. With waterless cookers take 2½ cups of water to 1 cup of rice. If the rice is prepared sweetened, add ½ cup of raisins and ½ cup of water.

THE PREPARATION OF LEGUMES

Legumes if properly prepared and used judiciously in the right quantity and combinations afford a pleasant change in the vegetarian dietary. They comprise the different varieties of beans, soy beans, peas, cow peas, chick peas (garbanzos), lentils, etc. Peanuts, on account of their chemical composition. are generally classed with the nuts. All legumes in their dry state require prolonged, slow cooking to render them thoroughly digestible and to bring out their rich flavors. Legumes should be steeped over night in distilled or soft water; some more water should be added before cooking in order to cover them well. Waterless Cookers and Savory Steam Double Boilers are very suitable for preparing legumes; waterless cookers develop a slight steam pressure. From 2 to 3 hours are generally necessary until the legumes are done. A fireless cooker may be used to advantage for this purpose. For many people the husks on the outer skin of the legumes are difficult of digestion. For this reason they should be rubbed through a colander, in order to remove most of the hulls. Legumes may also be ground into a flour by means of a nut mill; this also increases their digestibility and reduces the time of cooking. The addition of a little lemon juice and some vegetables and savory herbs also promotes their digestion. For the preparation of the ground legumes a Double Boiler is very appropriate.

There is a general opinion that legumes are valuable food for active hard-working people especially those who are much out of doors, but are not suited to those who take little exercise or to invalids. But even with indoor workers legumes will not cause distress in digestion if they are eaten in moderate amounts, not too often and in the right combinations. The amount taken at a meal should not exceed 4 ounces in the dry state or about 10 ounces when cooked. They should always be combined with green leaf vegetables, rich in sodium, such as celery, lettuce, chard, watercress, cabbage, etc. Legumes should not be eaten more than three times a week. In lumber and mining camps where beans are served almost daily and often combined with pork, the workers become afflicted with gout and rheumatism.

BOILED BEANS

½ lb. whole navy beans
1 pint water
2 tablespoons nut cream
1 teaspoon lemon juice
1 pinch salt

Soak the beans in the pint of water overnight and cook them in the morning until they are perfectly tender. Season with nut cream, lemon juice and salt if desired. Use a double boiler.

BAKED BEANS

½ lb. navy beans
1 pint water
2 tablespoons nut cream (peanut preferred)
1 teaspoon lemon juice

Soak the beans overnight, cook them in the morning until tender. Add the nut cream and lemon juice and bake in an oven for about 1 hour, stirring occasionally. When done, they should have rich brown color clear through.

STEWED LENTILS

1 cup lentils
2 cups water
¼ cup nut cream
1 teaspoon lemon juice
1 tablespoon chopped parsley

Wash the lentils well, soak them in the water overnight. In the morning cook them slowly for about 3 hours until they are soft and dry. When done add the nut cream, lemon juice and parsley. A chopped onion may be cooked with the lentils.

SIFTED LEGUMES

1 cup lentils, beans or peas
1½ cups water
3 tablespoons nut cream
1 teaspoon lemon juice

Soak the legumes in water overnight and slowly cook in the morning until tender. If all the water is absorbed add a little more hot water and put through a fine colander, taking a few tablespoons of the legumes at a time. When all sifted, add the nut cream and lemon juice and beat until smooth.

LENTIL LOAF

1 cup sifted lentils
1 cup bread crumbs; flaked legume cereal or some protein flour preferable
1 cup nut milk
1 tablespoon chopped parsley
½ teaspoon sage

Mix the ingredients well, put into well-oiled pan and bake in moderate oven until firm. Beans or peas may be substituted for lentils.

PUREES OF LEGUMES

Add sufficient nut milk to sifted beans, peas or lentils to make a thick batter and keep warm until ready to serve.

SAVORY GREEN PEAS

1 quart green peas
½ cup water
1 cup nut cream
1 tablespoon chopped parsley

Place the peas and water in the food pan of the Savory Double Boiler and cook until tender. Before serving add the nut cream and parsley.

LEGUME PATTIES

2 cups sifted legumes
1 cup flaked legume cereal or any preferred protein flour
1 beaten egg
1 tablespoon chopped parsley

Mix the ingredients and form into patties, about 2 inches wide and ½ inch thick. Bake for about 10 minutes and serve with nut cream and combination salad.

THE SOY BEAN, A REMARKABLE FOOD

The *soy bean,* also known as *soya* or *soya bean,* differs from most legumes in chemical composition but resembles the peanut, as it is rich both in protein and fat. About 20 varieties of the soy bean have been cultivated so far in the United States. They contain, on an average, 35 per cent protein, surpassing every other known vegetable in that respect, 20 per cent fat and very little starch. The carbohydrates, which amount to about 30 per cent, are found in the form of galactans, pentosan, sucrose, dextrin and cellulose. The mineral matter, as with in all seeds, principally consists of phosphate of potash, with appreciable quantities of magnesium, and a small amount of calcium and iron. It is deficient in sodium. Investigations show that the proportion of amino acids in the protein of the soy bean is not very different from that of meat proteins. In regard to its contents of the essential amino acids, the protein of the soy bean is superior to that of wheat and other cereals. It is often referred to as a vegetable casein as it is acted upon by strong acids and ferments and with these agents it yields the same product as does animal casein.

In Japan, China and northern India the soy bean largely takes the place of dairy products and meat. The great economical importance of the soy bean lies in the fact that seeds can be produced with less expense than those of any other leguminous crop, giving at the same time a larger yield, which ranges from 15 to 30 bushels per acre, according to the variety of the beans and condition of the soil. The soy bean is destined to become an important food product on the American continent, as it can be grown successfully through out the temperate zones. An interesting treatise on the soy bean has been recently published by Professors Charles Piper and William Morse from which some of the following data is taken.

In the Orient the soy bean is used in a great many ways. While the dry or mature beans can be satisfactorily prepared after the manner of navy or other beans, the immature or green soy beans, about three-fourths to full grown, make a most palatable and nutritious green vegetable, but the pods are too tough for this purpose. In order to remove the seeds quickly, they should be steamed in the pods for about 5 minutes. All through eastern Asia such products as soy bean flour, soy bean milk, soy bean cheese (tofu), soya sauce, soy bean oil, soy bean sprouts, etc., are used extensively. The soy bean and its products can now be bought in health food stores and in nearly all Japanese and Chinese grocery stores in cities having a large oriental population. The various methods of preparation of the soy bean are briefly given below.

BOILED SOY BEANS

The dry beans are best soaked in soft water over night or for at least 20 hours and then cooked with sufficient water in a waterless cooker or Pressure cooker until tender. This may require as much as 2 hours or more, according to the variety of beans used. The best results are obtained if the beans are allowed to simmer rather than boil quickly. Onions, tomatoes, celery, parsley and other seasoning vegetables increase the palatability of the soy bean. A fireless cooker may also be used in preparing soy beans for the table.

SOY BEAN MILK

Soy bean Milk has been drunk by the Orientals for over 2000 years. It is said to have been originated by the Chinese philosopher Whai Nain Tze, long before the Christian era. While mostly used in the fresh state by the Chinese it is also condensed like cow's milk by the Japanese. It also forms the basis of various kinds of vegetable cheese which are staple foods throughout Eastern Asia. Soy bean milk is best made by grinding the beans into fine flour. Take one cup of flour and add sufficient water to make a paste; then add 5 cups of boiling water and boil for 10 minutes in a double boiler, constantly stirring. When sufficiently cooled, filter through a cloth. The milky fluid obtained is rich in protein and fat, but deficient in lime, soda and salt. For this reason two or three tablespoons of spinach or carrot juice may be added to increase its alkalinity. The properties of the albuminous matter are similar to those of animal milk. Acids, rennet, pepsin and certain salt will cause coagulation of the protein. In China soy bean milk sweetened with sugar is taken as an early morning drink. It is extensively used throughout China for infant feeding, but for this purpose always a little fruit or vegetable juice and honey should be added. In many cities this vegetable milk is manufactured on a commercial scale and delivered in bottles to consumers each morning. In Japan a concentrated or condensed milk slightly sweetened, is made from the soy bean. A vacuum evaporater is best suited for this purpose.

TOFU

Tofu is made from soy beans by the addition of a small quantity of mineral salt or acid to the hot milk. A 1 percent solution of magnesium chlorid is generally used, in the ratio of about 1 part of solution to 4 parts of milk in order to produce coagulation of the plant casein. The Japanese usually add a 2 percent solution of concentrated seabrine, but lactic, tartaric and citric acid also give satisfactory results. The curds are separated by running the liquid through a cheese cloth and then are pressed into small cubes about 1 inch high.

Tofu is an easily digestible preparation of the soy bean; it is called by the Chinese "the meat without a bone." It contains 80 per cent water, 10 per cent protein. 4 per cent fat, 5 per cent carbohydrates and 1 per cent mineral matter. It is lacking however in alkaline elements and should therefore be eaten with vegetable salads. Tofu is also manufactured on a commercial scale and can be bought in most of the Japanese and Chinese grocery stores on the Pacific coast. Soy bean curd when freshly made is rather a tasteless product, but can be used as the basis of many preparations. It is frequently dried, after more water has been pressed out of it. Other preparations of the soy bean, which are but little known in this country are *natto, samananatto, Yuba and Miso.* The principal use of miso, which is a slightly fermented mixture of soy beans and rice or barley, is for making soups and in cooking vegetables.

SOY SAUCE

Soy sauce or shoyu which is a dark brown liquid with a rather pleasant odor and peculiar salty taste is made from a mixture of cooked and ground soy beans, parched and pulverized cereals, seabrine and water. This mixture is inoculated with a culture known as rice yeast and left in casks to ferment slowly from 6 to 12 months. Soy sauce is used daily by the Chinese and Japanese as a relish or condiment and its manufacture is an important industry all through Eastern Asia. The total production amounts to several million barrels annually. Soy sauce resembles in many respects the widely advertised extracts of brewers yeast, sold under various names as flavoring extracts. Soy sauce contains 62 per cent water, 9 per cent protein, 4 per cent glucose and dextrin and 20 per cent mineral matter of which 18 per cent is chloride of sodium or common salt. Soya sauce is a comparatively inexpensive article while the extracts of brewers yeast are sold at exorbitant prices. It may be used occasionally in small quantities for flavoring soups, stews and for countless other culinary needs.

SOY BEAN SPROUTS

Soy bean sprouts are used by the Chinese in considerable quantities as a green vegetable in a great variety of dishes. Bean sprouts furnish a fresh vegetable dish during the whole year, especially in winter when green vegetables are scarce or expensive. The dried beans are sprouted easily in a short time at the proper conditions of heat and moisture. After the beans are washed, they are placed in a wooden tub which has small holes in the bottom to drain off the excess of water which is poured over the beans. A bamboo mat or cloth is placed at the bottom of the vessel to prevent the beans from passing through the holes. The beans must be moistened at least three times daily in summer and twice in winter. In cold weather the beans should be kept warm and tepid water used for moistening the beans. The tub has to be covered with a heavy canvas to keep out the light. It takes about 3 days in summer and 2 weeks in winter until the sprouts are fully grown (1½ to 2 inches long) and ready to be eaten. Of the other varieties of beans the *mung bean* is best adapted for sprouting. It is more generally used for this purpose than is the soy bean, although the mung bean sprouts contain less protein, fat and mineral matter than do those of the soy bean. Bean sprouts are a wholesome inexpensive food and should be more extensively used, as they are rich in vitamins and make a delightful addition to combination salads.

BAKED SOY BEANS

2 cups soy beans, boiled according to directions given above
1 cup strained tomato pulp
1 tablespoon whole wheat flour
1 tablespoon chopped onions
1 tablespoon chopped parsley
1 dash of salt and paprika, if desired

Make a tomato sauce by mixing the flour and vegetables with the tomato pulp and heat until it thickens. Pour over the beans and bake in a moderately hot oven until brown.

SOY BEAN LOAF

2 cups boiled beans
1 cup flaked soy cereal; bread crumbs tolerable
1 cup chopped celery, steamed
½ cup chopped parsley
½ cup milk or nut milk
1 tablespoon whole wheat flour
1 teaspoon salt if desired

Mix the vegetables and flour with the milk and heat until it thickens, then mix thoroughly with the beans and flaked soy cereal. Form into a loaf of convenient shape and bake in an oiled pan until firm and brown. For Soy Bean Croquettes, brown onions in oil, mix with beans (mashed or riced) along with other ingredients, omitting milk or nut milk, if too fluidic, and mold into croquettes. Dip them slightly in beaten egg, then in corn meal, put in well-oiled shallow pans and bake until brown.

SOY BEAN BREAD

Part of the whole wheat flour and rye flour in the recipes given for bread can be substituted for soy bean flour. Not over one-third soy bean flour to two-thirds wheat or rye flour is suggested.

PEAS AND GARBANZOS

Sugar peas, which deserve to be better known, have an edible pod which is thicker and more fleshy than is the pod of the regular garden pea. The pods of the sugar pea are gathered when the seeds are just forming, and used, pod and all, exactly like string beans. Some varieties are excellent in flavor and texture if steamed until tender.

The *chick pea,* the *garbanzos* of Spain and Mexico, or the *gram* of India, contains less protein but more fat (about 6 per cent) than do the other legumes, except soy bean. Chick peas may be prepared like the other legumes, but they require a little longer boiling. If ground into flour they can be used for making soups and purees in the same way as are lentils and peas. The garbanzo is frequently roasted like peanuts and then ground into a meal.

Canned legumes, such as beans and peas, have become staple foods in America; they are cooked and hermetically sealed, to prevent fermentation. As long as they do not contain animal fat and are free from artificial coloring and preservatives they may be used occasionally during the winter season.

HOME MADE CHEESE

Man can live well without dairy products, if he makes judicious use of legumes and nuts in various forms, as has been shown in the preceding chapters, but under the present system of agriculture and production of food stuffs, many people have to make occasional use of milk products. As the commercial cheeses are generally heavily salted, preference should be given to home made cheeses.

Cheese should always be eaten with discrimination. It should never be used to top off an already substantial meal but should rather form an intrinsic part of the meal. The amount eaten daily should not exceed four ounces and all other protein foods, such as legumes or nuts should then be reduced. As cheese contains neither starch nor cellulose, it should be combined with a small amount of cereal products, succulent vegetables or fruits. One pound of cheese contains, on an average, 4 ounces of protein.

In the commercial manufacture of cheese the protein is precipitated by rennet, forming a curd which retains most of the fat. The curd is broken up, and the whole is heated to a temperature of about 100° F. The whey is drained off and carries with it most of the milk sugar, albumin and some of the organic salts, especially potassium, sodium and chlorine. The curd is salted, pressed and kept in a cool place for several weeks in order to "ripen" the cheese.

COTTAGE CHEESE

Cottage cheese made without salt is the most wholesome of cheeses. It is usually made by allowing the milk to sour naturally, although rennet is frequently used for the curdling process. The cheese made by rennet is milder in flavor and lacks the acid taste resulting from sour milk. The process of curdling the milk is hastened by keeping it at a temperature of 96° F, or blood heat. The curd is separated from the whey by means of a cheese cloth. As very little fat is retained in commercially manufactured cottage cheese, the addition of a little cream or nut cream makes it more palatable. Chopped parsley, onions, cloves or pimiento may be used for flavoring. Cottage cheese can be quickly made by using lemon juice for curdling the milk, according to the following method:

COTTAGE CHEESE MADE WITH LEMON JUICE

Use the juice of two medium sized lemons to one quart of milk. Put the milk and the strained lemon juice into earthenware or other non-aluminum pans and place in a gas ring with the flame turned low. An asbestos plate should be put between the pan and the gas flame, as the milk should not boil. When the curds are well separated from the whey, lay a piece of cheese cloth over a colander and pour in the contents of the pan. Gather up the corners of the cloth and hang up to drain for at least 15 minutes. Then place the cheese (still in the cloth) in the colander again and put a saucer with a weight on top. In about an hour the cheese will be ready. It will keep for two days in cold weather but must be made daily in warm weather.

SOUR CREAM CHEESE

Sour Cream Cheese is made like cottage cheese but requires no heating. The curd is formed either by souring or by the addition of rennet. If the cloth used for the curd is moistened by salt water, the whey will drain off easily.

COTTAGE CHEESE—FRENCH STYLE

This cheese is made from sour milk without heating; the sour milk is poured into earthen moulds which have small holes in the bottom. A fine sieve may take the place of the molds. After the whey is separated the curd will have a custard-like consistency. It makes a good combination with fruit, especially berries.

JUNKET

Junket is made from sweet milk and rennet, without breaking and separating the whey. It may be seasoned with a little cinnamon or grated nutmeg.

BULGARIAN BUTTERMILK

Bulgarian Buttermilk is made by using a special lactic acid ferment, the *bacillus bulgaricus.* In buttermilk, or in ordinary milk, which has been allowed to sour naturally, only about 1 per cent lactic acid is developed while the *bacillus bulgaricus* may carry fermentation to such a point that the milk may contain 2 per cent lactic acid or even more.

BUTTERMILK CREAM

Buttermilk Cream is a product which has been devised by the Wisconsin Experiment Station. By controlling the temperature in heating the buttermilk and not allowing it to go over 100° F, a compound is made which, after draining, has the consistency of a very thick cream. This cream may be used on bread in place of butter or as a salad dressing, or in combination with cereal dishes.

SALAD DRESSINGS

As salads are the most essential part of a rational diet, particular care should be given their preparation, especially to salad dressings. The nutritive and therapeutic value of salads is often ruined by the addition of vinegar and harsh spices. Vinegar is the product of acetic acid fermentation of alcohol and is a destroyer of red blood corpuscles. In many respects vinegar is worse than are the alcoholic liquors from which it is made and yet temperance reformers do not proscribe its use. The craving for vinegar and condiments is the result of perverted taste. All condiments have an irritating effect on the mucous membrane of the stomach and will retard proper digestion and assimilation. To the degree that we have acquired rational methods of eating all these condiments will become repulsive to us.

All salads should be made simply. There is no necessity of using a great many ingredients. Three or four kinds of vegetables should, as a rule, be sufficient. Fruits may be combined with green leaves and succulent vegetables, but not with starch-bearing roots. Salads should make the substantial part of at least one meal a day, they should constitute the principal dish and not be eaten as a mere supplement to a meal of starchy foods and meats.

Salads, if properly made, are great preservers of the alkalinity of the blood and are, therefore, indispensable for the preservation of our health. If they are eaten daily, even in winter time, there would be less tendency to "catch cold," which generally is the result of stuffing the body with artificial sweets, starches, fats and meats.

Instead of condiments we recommend powdered dehydrated kelp, powdered dehydrated sea lettuce (dulse), or any of the powdered dehydrated leafy vegetables, which are supplied in shakers for table use.

PLAIN SALAD DRESSING

4 tablespoons olive oil
2 tablespoons honey
2 tablespoons lemon juice
Mix thoroughly with an egg beater.

NUT BUTTER DRESSING

In addition to the plain Salad Dressing one or two tablespoons of nut cream may be added to each plate of salad. A recipe for making nut cream has been given above. Cream made from unroasted almond butter or peanut butter with the addition of a little honey is most suitable for salad dressing.

MAYONNAISE

Yolk of one egg
1 cup olive oil (7 ounces)
2 teaspoons lemon juice

Beat the yolk in a mixing bowl, adding some olive oil, drop by drop. When the mixture begins to thicken, alternately add a few drops of lemon juice and a few drops more oil until the desired consistency is obtained. Lemon juice thins the dressing, while the oil thickens it. If more lemon juice is added, oil must be added as the dressing should be stiff when ready to use.

FRENCH DRESSING

4 tablespoons olive oil
2 tablespoons lemon juice
A pinch of salt

The proportions of lemon juice and oil may be varied according to the ingredients of the salad and individual taste. Mix oil and salt by means of an egg beater and slowly add lemon juice.

FRENCH FRUIT DRESSING

4 tablespoons olive oil
3 tablespoons orange juice
3 tablespoons lemon juice
1 tablespoon honey

Mix ingredients with an egg beater.

WHIPPED CREAM DRESSING

4 tablespoons cream
1 tablespoon lemon juice
1 tablespoon honey

Whip cream and honey together and slowly add lemon juice. This makes a fine dressing for shredded lettuce, cold slaw, grated beets or some fruits.

SOUR CREAM DRESSING

1 cup sour cream
2 tablespoons honey
1 tablespoon lemon juice

Whip cream and honey together until thick; then slowly add lemon juice.

BANANA DRESSING

2 very ripe bananas
2 tablespoons nut cream
1 tablespoon honey
1 tablespoon lemon juice

Mash the bananas in a bowl with a spoon. Thoroughly mix the ingredients and let the finished dressing stand for 15 minutes before serving. This is an excellent dressing for salads.

PLAIN FRUIT DRESSING

2 tablespoons orange juice
2 tablespoons lemon juice
2 tablespoons of apple, grape or pineapple juice
1 tablespoon honey

Mix thoroughly.

ORANGE NUT DRESSING

Juice of 1 large ripe orange
1 tablespoon unroasted almond butter
1 teaspoon honey

Slowly add the orange juice to the almond butter and honey, thoroughly mixing the ingredients until the consistency of a smooth cream is obtained.

The following dairy products may also be used as salad dressings:

Cottage cheese
Sour cream cheese
Cottage cheese, French style
Buttermilk cream
(See recipes above)

COMBINATION VEGETABLE AND FRUIT SALADS

Salads are usually served in restaurants and homes as a side dish, badly prepared with vinegar and salt. Salads should form the larger portion of our meals; in fact, if made of the right ingredients, they almost constitute a wholesome nourishing meal in themselves with the addition of very little other food. The nutritive and hygienic value of green-leaf vegetables, succulent stems and roots has been repeatedly emphasized. In places and seasons when fresh fruits are scarce and expensive, vegetable salads should be eaten once or twice daily. Such vegetables as cabbage, carrots, pumpkins, turnips, onions, potatoes and many others may now be procured even in smaller towns during all seasons of the year.

No condiments whatsoever should enter into the preparation of vegetable salads, that is, if we want to derive full benefit from their regular use. Instead of using vinegar, pepper, mustard, salt, refined sugar, etc., either one or several of the following ingredients may be added in small quantities as flavoring: lemon juice, honey, grated horseradish, garlic, finely chopped leaves of mustard, sorrel, watercress, nasturtium, etc. The leaves of the flowers of dandelions, sweet peas, sweet clover, alfalfa, etc., may also be occasionally used for flavoring, as well as for decorative purposes. Combination salads should be made at least an hour before they are served, so that the different ingredients and flavors may blend together. The quantities given in the following recipes are about sufficient to make an ample portion for the average person. However, the amount given may be proportionately increased or decreased according to age and activity.

A good dish of combination salad with one of the hygienic dressings which have been described above and the addition of one or two slices of whole wheat bread, unleavened rye bread, or a baked potato, make up a most wholesome and nourishing meal. Salads should be eaten daily by adults and also by children, as soon as their teeth are sufficiently developed to masticate thoroughly their food. Leafy vegetables and tender roots supply the most essential and wholesome food constituents which keep the blood in an alkaline condition and are, therefore, nature's truly preventive medicine. Cultivate the salad habit and save doctor bills.

In the United States, because of its large territory, and our improved methods of transportation, a large variety of fresh vegetables can be obtained during all seasons. The following varieties may be purchased in the larger markets almost any month of the year.

Beets
Cabbage
Carrots
Cauliflower
Celery
Endive
Garlic
Horseradish
Kohlrabi
Lettuce
Mushrooms
Onions
Peppers
Potatoes
Pumpkins
Radishes
Romaine Lettuce
Spinach
Tomatoes
Turnips
Vegetable Marrow
Watercress
Yams

VEGETABLE SALADS

(See recipes for dressings on pages 180 to 182)

COMBINATION No. 1

1 small head of lettuce
1 small bunch of celery
2 large carrots
2 tablespoons plain salad dressing
2 tablespoons nut cream

Wash and clean the vegetables, cut the lettuce and celery into small pieces and grate the carrots. Mix the vegetables, with the plain salad dressing. When ready to serve, dress with nut cream.

COMBINATION No. 2

1 small head lettuce
2 medium-sized tomatoes
1 turnip
1 small onion
½ cup Sour Cream Dressing

Slice lettuce, tomatoes and the onion, grate turnips, mix the vegetables together and dress with sour cream.

COMBINATION No. 3

½ head cabbage
3 stalks celery
Some endive
½ cup Whipped Cream Dressing

Run the vegetables through a food chopper and apply dressing.

COMBINATION No. 4

½ head cabbage
2 medium-sized apples
1 cup Banana Dressing

Chop and mix the ingredients and apply dressing.

COMBINATION No. 5

1 small head lettuce
½ bunch watercress
4 green onions
2 tablespoons Plain Salad Dressing
4 ounces cottage cheese

Chop the ingredients fine and mix with the plain Dressing and serve with cottage cheese.

COMBINATION No. 6

½ bunch spinach
½ bunch watercress
2 carrots
2 tablespoons mayonnaise

Wash and clean the vegetables; run them through the fine knife of a food chopper and serve on lettuce leaves with mayonnaise.

COMBINATION No. 7

2 medium-sized carrots
½ head lettuce
1 small onion
½ cup Sour Cream Dressing

Grate the carrots and cut the onion into slices about ¼ inch thick, lay them on lettuce leaves and decorate with asparagus, which may be slightly steamed. Apply dressing.

COMBINATION No. 8

2 medium-sized tomatoes
6 stalks celery
1 green pepper
½ cup grated nuts
2 tablespoons French Dressing

Slice the tomatoes, remove the seeds from the pepper and the tough fibres from the celery. Cut the pepper and celery into small pieces and put on lettuce leaves together with tomatoes. Cover with the nut meal and dressing.

COMBINATION No. 9

1 large cucumber
1 doz. small radishes
1 small head cauliflower, steamed or raw
2 tablespoons Plain Salad Dressing
2 tablespoons nut butter dressing

Slice the cucumber and the radishes and cut the cauliflower into flowerets, Mix the vegetables with the plain dressing and serve on lettuce leaves with nut butter dressing.

COMBINATION No. 10

2 potatoes (medium size)
1 cucumber
1 onion
3 stalks celery
Some minced parsley
1 cup buttermilk cream

Peel the potatoes and steam in Savory Double Boiler for about 40 minutes. Slice the potatoes, cucumber and onion. Cut the celery into small pieces and dress with buttermilk cream.

COMBINATION No. 11

2 medium-sized cucumbers
2 medium-sized tomatoes
2 small onions (Bermuda, if obtainable)
1 sprig parsley
2 tablespoons mayonnaise

Peel the cucumbers, slice all the vegetables and dress with mayonnaise.

COMBINATION No. 12

2 cups string beans, cut fine
½ head lettuce
1 cup watercress, chopped fine
1 bunch small radishes, cut fine
1 Bermuda onion, sliced
2 tablespoons Plain Salad Dressing
4 ounces cottage cheese

Steam the string beans in the Savory Double Boiler and mix with the vegetables and Plain Dressing.

COMBINATION No. 13

½ head lettuce, cut into small pieces
1 cup diced celery (about 5 stalks or 4 ounces)
2 sliced bananas (6 ounces)
1 grated apple (6 ounces)
½ cup almond cream

Mix the ingredients together and dress with almond cream.

COMBINATION No. 14

2 medium-sized tomatoes
1 medium-sized cucumber
6 small radishes
½ sweet green pepper
2 tablespoons French Dressing
½ cup chopped nuts

Slice the tomatoes, cucumbers and radishes and arrange nicely on lettuce leaves. Chop the green pepper and sprinkle on top of the other vegetables. Then add the salad dressing and chopped nuts.

COMBINATION No. 15

1 cup grated carrots
½ cup grated turnips
1 cup diced potatoes
1 cup string beans, cut small
½ cup Sour Cream Dressing

Steam the potatoes and string beans in the Savory Double Boiler until soft (about ½ hour), let them cool and then mix with the other vegetables. Pour the dressing over and serve.

COMBINATION No. 16

¼ head cabbage
2 carrots
1 oz. seedless raisins
2 bananas
4 stalks celery
1 tablespoon honey
½ cup nut butter dressing

Grate the cabbage and carrots; slice the bananas and celery, add the honey, raisins and nut butter dressing.

COMBINATION No. 17

3 medium-sized carrots
6 to 8 stalks celery
1 large onion
1 tablespoon Plain Salad Dressing
4 ounces cottage cheese

Grate the carrots, run celery and onion through a food chopper; mix all ingredients and serve on lettuce leaves.

COMBINATION No. 18

2 medium-sized carrots (1 cup grated)
1 cup new peas (raw or steamed)
1 cup spinach chopped fine (raw)
1 tablespoon chopped onions or chives
1 tablespoon parsley
2 tablespoons French Salad Dressing

Thoroughly mix all ingredients.

COMBINATION No. 19

1 cup pitted ripe olives
1 cup chopped watercress
6 stalks celery, cut into small pieces
1 green sweet pepper
6 small green onions
2 tablespoons mayonnaise

Wash celery and onions and cut into small pieces, chop pepper, removing seeds and white pith, blend altogether and dress with mayonnaise.

COMBINATION No. 20

1 large ear sweet corn
¼ head cabbage
2 stalks celery
1 medium-sized onion
½ cup nut cream

Shell the corn and run all the ingredients through food chopper. If desired, steam in Savory Double Boiler for 30 minutes. Dress with nut cream or Sour Cream Dressing.

COMBINATION No. 21

½ head red cabbage
2 medium-sized carrots
watercress
3 stalks celery
2 tablespoons plain salad dressing
2 tablespoons nut cream

Grate carrots; run cabbage and celery through food chopper, and mix with the plain Salad Dressing. Serve on watercress with nut cream.

COMBINATION No. 22

1 medium-sized avocado (about 6 ounces)
½ head lettuce
½ bunch spinach
3 stalks celery
1 cup Banana Dressing

Pit avocado and cut into slices; chop lettuce, celery and spinach, mix ingredients together and apply dressing.

COMBINATION No. 23

½ bunch spinach
3 stalks celery
1 small head cauliflower, steamed if preferred
2 tablespoons mayonnaise

Chop the spinach and celery fine; remove stem from cauliflower and cut into small pieces or flowerets and serve on lettuce leaves with mayonnaise.

COMBINATION No. 24

1 large Chinese radish
2 medium-sized carrots (1 cup)
½ head lettuce
4 stalks celery
2 tablespoons Plain Salad Dressing
4 ounces cottage cheese or powdered soy milk creamed with water

Grate the radish and carrots, chop lettuce and celery; add salad dressing and cottage cheese or soy milk and thoroughly mix all ingredients.

COMBINATION No. 25

2 cups bean sprouts
1 tomato
¼ head cabbage
4 stalks celery
1 onion
½ cup Sour Cream Dressing

Slice the tomato; chop cabbage, celery and onion; blend ingredients together and apply Sour Cream Dressing.

COMBINATION No. 26

10 stalks asparagus
1 small head cauliflower, steamed if preferred
3 stalks celery
2 medium size tomatoes
1 Bermuda onion
2 tablespoons mayonnaise

Cut into small pieces the tender portions of asparagus, break the cauliflower into flowerets, slice tomatoes, celery and onions and arrange ingredients on plates covered with lettuce leaves. Dress with mayonnaise.

COMBINATION No. 27

2 carrots
1 turnip
1 bunch green onions
1 cup chopped watercress or dandelion leaves
2 tablespoons Plain Salad Dressing
4 ounces cottage cheese

Grate carrots and turnips, chop watercress and lower parts of onions; blend ingredients together with Plain Salad Dressing. Serve on lettuce leaves with cottage cheese.

COMBINATION No. 28

1 small head endive or ½ head cabbage
2 carrots
2 stalks celery
2 bananas
2 tablespoons Plain Salad Dressing
2 tablespoons nut butter dressing

Cut fine the endive or cabbage; grate the carrots and apples, mix the Plain Dressing and vegetables together and cover with sliced bananas. When ready serve on lettuce leaves and cover with the nut butter dressing.

COMBINATION No. 29

1 cup grated carrots
1 cup chopped spinach
1 cup chopped Swiss chard
½ bell pepper chopped fine
3 stalks celery cut fine
1 tablespoon chopped parsley
½ cup Sour Cream Dressing

Thoroughly mix the ingredients and apply dressing.

COMBINATION No. 30

1 slice pumpkin, raw, peeled and grated
1 cup grated beets
1 cup chopped watercress
2 tablespoons Plain Salad Dressing
½ cup nut butter dressing

Mix the vegetables and salad dressing, serve on lettuce leaves with nut cream.

COMBINATION No. 31

1 cup grated parsnips
1 cup grated carrots
½ head lettuce grated fine
3 stalks celery cut fine
2 tablespoons mayonnaise

Mix the ingredients and dress with mayonnaise.

COMBINATION No. 32

1 cup bean sprouts
1 cup grated carrots
½ head Romaine lettuce cut fine
2 tablespoons Plain Salad Dressing
4 ounces cottage cheese, or soy bean butter or soy cheese

Mix the vegetables with the plain dressing and serve on lettuce leaves with cottage cheese or soy cheese.

FRUIT SALADS

FRUIT SALAD IN ORANGE CUPS No. 33

3 oranges
2 slices pineapple, cubed
½ cup seedless raisins
2 tablespoons nut butter dressing

Cut oranges in two; carefully remove pulp, then pull out all membranes, leaving orange cups. Mix pineapple and raisins with the orange pulp and fill orange cups. Cover with nut cream and serve on lettuce leaves.

CALIFORNIA FRUIT SALAD No. 34

1 medium-sized avocado
1 grapefruit
3 oranges

Peel and slice avocado and moisten with lemon juice. Peel grapefruit and oranges and remove pulp from membrane. Arrange the three kinds of fruit on salad plates covered with head lettuce and serve with Orange Nut Dressing. (See Salad Dressings.)

TROPICAL FRUIT SALAD No. 35

2 oranges
3 ripe bananas
1 avocado
4 slices pineapple, cubed
1 dozen brazil nuts, grated

Peel and slice fruit; mix all ingredients and serve as above. Plain almond cream also goes well with the salad.

RAISIN AND CELERY SALAD No. 36

1 small bunch celery
2 apples
1 cup seedless raisins
1 cup grated nuts

Cut apples and celery into small pieces or run through the coarse knife of food chopper. Mix all ingredients, serve on lettuce leaves and moisten with Plain Salad Dressing.

NECTARINE SALAD No. 37

4 nectarines, cut in small pieces
½ basket raspberries or loganberries
1 dozen cherries

Stem and pit the cherries, mix the fruit together and serve on lettuce leaves with the Nut Cream Dressing. Three large peaches or 6 large apricots may be used instead of nectarines.

PEAR SALAD No. 38

2 Russet or Bartlett pears
1 apple
2 medium-sized oranges

Cut the fruit into small pieces and dress with 2 tablespoons nut cream. Serve on lettuce leaves.

BERRY AND BANANA COMBINATION No. 39

3 ripe bananas
1 basket berries (8 ounces) in season
¼ cup nut cream
1 tablespoon honey

Peel the bananas, wash the berries and mash fruit and nut cream in a suitable bowl.

COMBINATION No. 40

½ cantaloupe peeled and cut into small pieces
2 slices pineapple, cut fine
1 small basket raspberries or blackberries
½ cup nut butter dressing or banana dressing

Mix the fruits and celery together, put on lettuce leaves and dress with nut cream or banana dressing.

APPLE AND ORANGE COMBINATION No. 41

2 juicy apples
2 ripe bananas
1 ripe orange
½ cup of almond cream or peanut cream

Peel and slice the fruit, and proceed as above.

CHERRY AND BANANA COMBINATION No. 42

1 pound cherries
2 ripe bananas
½ cup nut cream

Pit the cherries; peel and slice the bananas and proceed as above.

APRICOT AND BANANA COMBINATION No. 43

1 lb. apricots
2 ripe bananas
½ cup nut cream

Pit the apricots and cut them into quarters; peel and slice the bananas and proceed as above.

PEACH AND MELON COMBINATION No. 44

1 lb. peaches
½ cantaloupe or 1 slice of cassaba melon
½ cup nut cream or Orange Nut Dressing

Peel and slice the peaches; scoop out the cantaloupe or cassaba in small pieces by means of a teaspoon and proceed as above.

STUFFED CELERY No. 45

Wash and clean celery stalks and fill the groove of each stalk with nut butter or pimento cottage cheese. Stuffed celery may be eaten with any of the fruit salads.

SUNSHINE SALAD

Peel and slice crosswise firm, medium-sized oranges, allowing four or five slices for each salad. Dip orange slices in warm honey (both sides) then in cocoanut. Arrange on nested crisp lettuce. Heap fresh berries in the center where orange slices meet, drizzle a bit of honey about the fruit, and serve cold.

If you read a recipe suggesting "drizzling" the honey, remember that cold honey is thick and does not spread easily or well, but warm honey does and blends nicely; place the jar or dish of honey in warm, not hot, water for about ten minutes before using, then the honey will be in the right consistency to make tiny permeating threads, instead of thick streams.

WHY ABSTINENCE FROM FLESH FOODS IS ADVOCATED

Arguments in Favor of Meat-Eating

No recipes are given in this book for the preparation of meats. It has been proven conclusively that we can select from the various products of the vegetable kingdom a complete and satisfactory diet, superior in every respect to the so-called mixed diet. This fact is becoming more and more acknowledged now by leading physiologists. Of course, there are still persons who, being financially interested in cattle raising and meat-packing, are promulgating all kinds of false and misleading arguments to persuade people to "eat more meat."

This is done to keep their industries on a paying basis. Their advertising campaign is carried on from a merely commercial point of view.

Because a habit is time honored does not prove that it is right. The slaughter of millions of animals every year for human food is as unnecessary as it is cruel and wasteful. Those who cannot altogether dispense with meat for some reason may occasionally partake of fresh fish, as the lesser of two evils, but the fact remains that the various proteins of the vegetable kingdom furnish us with all the necessary amino acids without the waste products which are contained in the muscular tissues or glandular organs of the animal.

The principal argument in favor of meat-eating is that animal protein is more easily digested than is vegetable protein. This may be true, but it has been shown that for the final reconstructive processes of our bodily cells flesh foods are inadequate; they are deficient in the blood, bone and tissue building elements, while their proteins are lacking in certain amino acids. Carnivorous animals partake of every part of their prey, blood, bones, tendons, cartilages, viscera, etc. The Eskimos, who largely live on meat and fat, instinctively preserve the blood of the slaughtered animals, in order to supply themselves with the alkaline bases contained in the blood.

Because a certain food or food principle is quickly absorbed by the digestive tract does not indicate its superior nutritive value. Food products made from white flour and refined sugar may be more easily digested than are some of the coarser foods made from the whole grain and fruits, but we know that the former starve the nerves and tissues, and in time, create serious digestive disturbances.

Meat, a Stimulant

The idea that we must eat meat in order to keep up our bodily strength was advanced by some of the earlier physiologists, like Liebig and Voit, who believed that meat makes meat, that by eating the muscular tissues of animals we could build strong muscles. Of course this false idea has been scientifically refuted long ago, but it is still prevalent among the masses. We cannot increase our muscular strength and endurance by meat eating any more than we can improve our mental capacity by a daily ration of calves' brains. Man's physical and mental powers have been developed in the long struggle for existence during millions of years; they can only be improved by constantly exercising them and not by eating specific foods. Meat, like all foods, has a certain stimulating effect, which is due largely to the amount of waste products it contains. We can stimulate our nervous system by a number of poisonous alkaloidal substances, resembling those contained in meat, like thein, caffein, nicotin, etc., but this stimulation does not add anything to our nerve power. To the contrary, it depletes our reserve forces. A man may have the feeling of bodily warmth and strength after a meal of meat, but the fact is that the digestion of flesh foods wears out the stomach and kidneys prematurely, by increasing the acidity of the blood and by the accumulation of toxins in the system. As a result we see men dying of arteriosclerosis, heart failure, apoplexy, Bright's disease, cancer, etc., at ages of from fifty to sixty years, and sometimes earlier, when they should be at the very height of mental and physical vigor and be most useful to their fellow men.

The Importance of Diet Reform

We realize, however, that meat will be a staple food for many years to come, partly because the majority of people are slow in changing their habits of eating and partly because the meat industry with all its ramifications is so closely interwoven with the present social and economic system that any sudden and radical change in the methods of living of the great masses is hardly probable. The general adoption of more rational methods of living depends to a great extent on the establishment of an educational system which will take better care of the physical, mental and moral welfare of the rising generation.

Diet reform is more or less an individual problem and naturally goes on slowly, but it is the author's belief that if people were given the right information, instead of almost daily presented with all kinds of erroneous and misleading statements in regard to foods and nutrition, they would change their methods of living more rapidly than they do now. Our dietetic habits are acquired in early childhood. Children, if not influenced by the habits of their parents and teachers, will always prefer the natural products of the soil to meat. Young people will find no difficulty in giving up meat if they are taught how to select and combine their foods for the purpose of building strong and healthy bodies.

Those who are past middle life and have eaten meat twice or three times daily are apt not to give up meat suddenly, but they can gradually wean themselves from the habit by first eating meat only once daily and then not oftener than twice or three times weekly. At any rate, the quantity eaten daily should not exceed four ounces and should be combined with a dish of combination salad, in order to facilitate the elimination of waste poisons. By the proper use of nuts, unroasted nut butters and occasionally legumes or dairy products, if vegetable proteins are not available, we can secure all the necessary protein and amino acids, in much better and purer form than those which occur in flesh foods. In a more enlightened society meat will be entirely discarded from the dietary, for economical and hygienic as well as moral reasons. Meat-eating is one of the greatest economic wastes and the cause of much ill health while the slaughtering of animals perpetuates cruelty and crime. We call many of the undomesticated animal "beasts of prey." If those beasts of prey could speak, what would they call us?

It is well-known that one of the outstanding features of the average American dinner table is the great variety of dishes served at the same meal. This is not only a great waste of time and food materials, but also leads to overeating and to impairment of health. We should realize that we not only prevent disease by incorporating into each meal a limited natural variety, but that such a diet, if judiciously chosen, will also increase our physical and mental efficiency. It is to simplicity of diet that we should look for redemption of our bodily ills. By living on natural and wholesome foods, derived largely if not entirely from the vegetable kingdom, we shall find that we can do a great amount of constructive work on a comparatively small amount of food, while by the consumption of meat, spices, condiments, alcohol, tobacco, etc., we dissipate our vital forces in a selfish and useless manner. By reforming our dietetic habits we shall, therefore, not only benefit ourselves, but also increase our usefulness to mankind and make an important stride toward the solution of all our social and economic problems.

CHAPTER XX

RATIONAL FOOD COMBINATIONS

Specific Dietetic Rules

The menus outlined in this chapter are divided into three daily meals. Three meals are most convenient for the majority of people. They provide about 2,000 calories, consisting of 1½ ounces of protein, 12 ounces of carbohydrates, 2 ounces of fat and an adequate amount of cellulose and organic salts—altogether from 16 to 18 ounces of water-free substance. These amounts can be increased or decreased proportionately, according to age, occupation and climatic conditions. For small children and very old people the amounts should be reduced about one to one-half. There is little danger of overeating on simple natural foods, free from condiments and spices which tickle our palate and misguide our appetite. The following dietetic rules should be observed:

Eat only when hungry and not because it is breakfast or lunch time.

Eat slowly; masticate every morsel. Enjoy your food and do not harbor any disagreeable thoughts while eating. Make your repast as pleasant as possible.

Eat without drinking. This insures thorough mastication and insalivation and also helps to preserve the teeth. In hot weather begin your meal with fresh juicy fruit; you will find that very little else is needed.

Do not take very hot or very cold foods or drinks. Ice water and hot soups have ruined many stomachs. If a liquid such as water or cereal drink is desired it should be taken at least ½ hour after the meal or before eating.

If anything is desired between meals, a little juicy fruit may be eaten.

Fruit juices, milk or buttermilk should be sipped slowly and not gulped down hastily. Remember that they are foods not drinks as a rule; fruits and vegetables are best eaten at separate meals; occasionally, however, one or two kinds of fruit may be combined with leafy vegetables in the form of combination salads, but underground vegetables and fruits should not be eaten together.

Do not, as a general practice, eat more than one kind of starch at the same meal.

It is best not to combine starchy foods and fruits. although there are some people with good digestions who can eat cereal foods and sub-acid fruits together without any ill effects.

No more than two or three kinds of foods should be eaten at the same meal. There may, however, be a variety of compatible fruits or vegetables.

The *mono-diet,* that is, eating only one kind of food at a time, often produces good results, especially with people whose digestive organs are not very strong. The kind of food can be changed from meal to meal, so that monotony is avoided. Each food has its own cellular vibration; and in order to derive the full benefit from natural products, fruits particularly, they should be eaten alone to allow their vibratory forces to exert their full potency. By living on a mono-diet, which should consist largely of fruits, the food constituents are more completely utilized than is the case when subsisting on a mixed diet, while a large amount of nerve force is conserved in the process of digestion. All animals in the natural state practically live on a mono-diet. This, to a large extent, accounts for their superb health, wonderful agility and freedom from disease. Domesticated animals, that have lost their natural instincts and have acquired abnormal eating habits, are subject to the same ailments as is man.

Vital Economy in the Use of Foods

The daily amount of food needed has been so far a matter of controversy among dietitians. It has been shown how we can safely reduce the amount of protein, by eating foods rich in alkaline elements. By living mostly on natural, uncooked foods (fruits, green leaf vegetables, and nuts) we can get along with a much smaller amount of food, measured according to calories, than when living on cooked and acid-forming foods. In the former case the foods are much better utilized and supply a relatively much larger amount of material for repairing tissues and producing vital energy, than do artificially prepared and devitalized foods. A man may, therefore, be starving on 4000 calories per day and be well nourished on 2000 calories per day. Through years of experiments on his body, as well as by directing the diet of others, the author has found that the average person may live well on 2000 calories per day, provided the foods are judiciously selected, so they give a maximum amount of energy, with the least expenditure of nerve force in digestion, assimilation and elimination of waste products.

How to Increase Endurance

In case of prolonged hard muscular work the amounts should be proportionately increased. If we use 1 ounce (equal to 113 calories) more of protein foods, we should correspondingly increase the amount of fruits or vegetables by about 300 calories in order to preserve the alkalinity of the blood and to lessen the effect of the fatigue poisons. The wonderful feats of endurance performed by vegetarian athletes are the result of their strongly alkaline diet, which insures the rapid elimination of the waste poisons which, if too long retained in the system, soon cause fatigue. Intense and continued brain work is likewise favored by a more or less exclusive fruit diet. Of course, there are those who are prone to stimulate their mental activities by the use of tobacco, alcoholic beverages, coffee, tea and sometimes by highly seasoned meats, but in all these cases the body lives on its reserve forces and finally the nervous system becomes exhausted. The continued use of stimulants and narcotics usually leads to a complete nervous breakdown. This is often ascribed to overwork, but is really the result of artificial stimulation and the accumulation of toxins in blood and tissues.

It is well to remind the reader that normal alkaline blood can only be formed when the proportion of the base-forming to the acid-forming foods (according to the amount of water free substance or calories), is at least two to one, or still better three to one as is explained as follows.

HOW TO PROPORTION AND REGULATE OUR MEALS

In the selection and combination of our foods we should first of all see that we get a sufficiency of the alkaline elements. The amount of calories, while useful as a purely quantitative measure, should be only of secondary importance. If, for instance, the daily food requirement of a man at moderate muscular work amounts to about 2100 calories—equal to about 20 ounces of water-free substance, at least 1400 calories should be furnished in the form of fruits and vegetables and 700 calories in the form of nuts, cereal foods, legumes and dairy products. These figures are of course only approximate, as no absolute rules in regard to the quantity of food can be made. As a guide, however, we may accept the following amounts of calories needed in each instance.

Man at hard muscular work	2600-2700	calories
Man at moderate muscular work	2100-2200	"
Man at light muscular work and boys 15 and 16 years old	2000	"
Man at sedentary occupation, woman at moderately active work	1800	"
Woman at light work and boys and girls 12 to 14 years old	1550-1600	"
Boys and girls 10 to 12 years old	1350-1400	"
Children, 6 to 9 years old	1100	"
Children, 2 to 5 years old	875- 900	"
Children, under 2 years old	650	"

In the case of a man at moderate muscular work, the daily dietary should consist of:

From 2 to 3 pounds of fresh fruits, if dried fruits are taken the amount should be reduced accordingly. Four ounces of dried fruit are about equal to one pound of fresh fruit; altogether about 900 calories.

From 1 to 1½ pounds of leafy vegetables, succulent roots and bulbs, starchy roots and tubers, after they are cleaned and trimmed, altogether about 500 calories.

From 4 to 6 ounces of whole wheat bread, which is about equal in calories to a large cup of boiled rice or a large baked potato with butter; each about 350 calories.

From 2 to 3 ounces of nuts or unroasted nut butter, this is equivalent in protein contents to 4 ounces cottage cheese, or to a large cup of boiled legumes (about 8 ounces), or 3 eggs; each about 350 calories.

Perhaps it will sometimes be impossible to strictly adhere to this outlined regimen, as we may be in places where an ideal diet cannot be procured. But in the selection and combination of our food we should always be careful to preserve the alkalinity of the blood. Even in northern countries some kind of vegetables like cabbage, carrots, potatoes, turnips, etc. can be bought during the winter months, while such fresh fruits as apples, bananas, oranges, and dried fruits like figs, dates, prunes and raisins are available almost everywhere during all seasons of the year.

The secret of maintaining our normal bodily weight is found in the alkalinity of our diet. In case of thin and anemic people, it improves the quality of the blood and increases the strength of the digestive juices, thus working gradually towards better assimilation and normal tissue building; while in the case of obese persons it brings about better oxidation and elimination of waste matter and reduction of adipose tissue. In either case, however, deep breathing and moderate exercise in the open air greatly help to attain the desired results.

CHAPTER XXI

SIMPLE AND WELL-BALANCED MENUS FOR ALL SEASONS

The Importance of Simplicity in Eating

The following menus serve as a useful guide for the proper selection and combination of foods and may be slightly changed to utilize the products of the seasons in different localities. They provide a sufficiency of alkaline elements, mostly in the form of natural uncooked foods. A number of menus is given made up entirely of uncooked foods. As precisely mentioned they furnish on an average about 2000 calories per day. In case of hard muscular work the amounts of fruits, nuts and cereals should be increased proportionately. But we shall find that a much smaller quantity of food is needed to appease hunger after the organism has been freed of encumbrances, with stored up debris effectively uprooted by strongly eliminative natural measures; and a regenerated and remineralized blood stream rendered more alkaline. Thus vital nourishment finds its way unimpeded to life-sustaining nerve centers and glands. Equally important, the ordinary mixed diet, consisting of much artificially prepared and denatured foods makes it necessary for us to consume a greater amount of food to satisfy physiological needs. By adhering to a simple and rational diet, the strength of our digestive juices increases, the food we eat is better utilized and the waste matter quickly eliminated; we are able to work longer and think more clearly with less fatigue, than if our blood is overloaded with toxins, arising from overeating and drug stimulation. At the same time it is a less arduous task for us to control our emotions and become masters of ourselves.

Drinking with meals should be avoided as much as possible. It is much better to take water or cereal drinks at least an hour after a meal. If we discard salt and pepper from our dietary, the desire for drinking will be greatly reduced. Meat, white flour, refined sugar, spices and vinegar have been excluded. The use of dairy products has been reduced to a minimum; they have been replaced largely by nuts, nut products and legumes properly prepared. Those who are not ready to accept fully the menus as outlined should at least attempt to adhere to them as closely as possible. But we must recognize that the fundamental cause of the thousand and one diseases named in medical dictionaries is the toxemic condition of blood and tissues due to wrong eating, thinking and living. Hence the following food combinations will prove of invaluable assistance in solving one of the greatest problems confronting mankind—the prevention and cure of disease.

All the menus have been arranged according to the recipes in the preceding chapter. The amounts of the ingredients in the respective recipes for combination salads, including dressings, represent an average portion for an adult person. The foods have been selected according to seasons. People who live in subtropical climates can get fresh vegetables and fruits all the year around at reasonable prices, or if they are fortunate enough to raise them in their own gardens. None the less, by means of our improved methods of transportation, we can now procure in the northern temperate zone many kinds of fresh vegetables and fruits during the winter. Unsulphured dried fruits, nuts and unroasted nut butters supply a maximum of heat and energy with the least expenditure of vital force. Even in cold climates a man can maintain very well health and vitality with a plentiful supply of dried fruits, cereals, legumes, nut butters and nuts, supplemented by such vegetables as can be easily procured.

Simplicity in eating must be the keynote in the attainment of lasting mental and physical health; it is one of the greatest factors in the conservation of vital force and in the prolongation of life.

WINTER MENUS

No. 1 (Monday)

Breakfast

1 orange
5 ounces dried prunes (soaked in water for 24 hours and warmed in the morning)
Dressed with 2 tablespoons nut cream

Lunch

Combination salad No. 1
2 slices whole wheat bread (4 ounces)

Dinner

1 large baked potato (8 ounces) with butter
1 bunch spinach or kale, 6 stalks celery, 1 carrot, 1 onion, cut fine and steamed in the Savory Double Boiler
Dressed with 2 tablespoons nut cream or 1 egg

No. 2 (Tuesday)

Breakfast

½ grapefruit with teaspoon honey
5 oz. dried black figs (soaked in water over night and warmed in the morning)
Dressed with 2 tablespoons nut cream

Lunch

Combination salad No. 2 with sour cream dressing
A few stalks of celery stuffed with soy butter
A few sun-dried olives

Dinner

1 plate boiled beans (6 ounces)
1 plate cold slaw (8 ounces) with 2 tablespoons Plain Salad Dressing and 2 tablespoons mayonnaise
Few stalks celery or ½ head lettuce may accompany cold slaw
½ egg plant, buttered

No. 3 (Wednesday)

Breakfast

1 ripe banana sliced
2 baked apples dressed with 2 tablespoons nut cream

Lunch

Combination salad No. 3 with whipped cream dressing
2 slices whole wheat bread

Dinner

1 plate vegetable soup
½ head lettuce
2 cups boiled whole rice
Dressed with 2 tablespoons nut cream or flaxseed meal immersed in hot water and vegetable extract

No. 4 (Thursday)

Breakfast

½ grapefruit with teaspoon honey
5 ounces Calimyrna Figs (soaked in water over night and warmed in the morning); dressed with 2 tablespoons nut cream

Lunch

Combination salad No. 4
A few nut meats or ½ avocado

Dinner

1 plate celery soup with whole wheat crackers
2 slices spinach nut loaf (8 to 10 ounces) with tomato dressing
A few ripe olives
A side dish of cold slaw

No. 5 (Friday)

Breakfast

1 orange
5 ounces unsulphured dried apricots soaked in water over night and warmed in the morning
Dressed with 2 tablespoons nut cream

Lunch

Combination salad No. 5, with French Dressing and cottage cheese
A few steamed, buttered and sliced beet roots or parsnips if relished

Dinner

1 plate bean soup
1 bunch spinach, 2 sliced carrots and 2 onions steamed in a double boiler
2 tablespoons nut cream as dressing or 1 egg
Side dish of sliced raw rutabagas, celery stalks

No. 6 (Saturday)

Breakfast

½ grapefruit with teaspoon honey
5 ounces unsulphured dried pears soaked in water over night and dressed with 2 tablespoons nut cream

Lunch

Combination salad No. 6
2 slices whole wheat bread or 2 corn and potato muffins

Dinner

1 plate onion and potato soup
Combination salad No. 29

No. 7 (Sunday)

Breakfast

1 orange
5 ounces unsulphured dehydrated peaches soaked in water over night and warmed in the morning; dressed with 2 tablespoons nut cream

Lunch

Combination salad No. 7
Dressed with ½ cup sour-cream or nut cream
A small dish of whole wheat spaghetti, plain or with just a dash of cheese; butter; or flaxseex meal immersed in hot water and flavored with vegetable extract; or mushroom sauce

Dinner

1 plate cream of tomato soup
2 slices nut loaf served on lettuce leaves, dressed with banana sauce (see recipes)
3 stalks celery stuffed with finely minced vegetables, blended with nut cream or mayonnaise
A few sun-dried olives

SPRING MENUS

No. 8 (Monday)

Breakfast

½ grapefruit with teaspoon honey
2 baked apples with 2 tablespoons nut cream
1 ripe banana

Lunch

Combination Salad No. 8 with French Dressing
A slice of baked Hubbard squash

Dinner

1 plate lentil soup
Spinach or kale, mustard greens and onions, steamed in the Double Boiler, creamed with two tablespoons flaxseed meal and vegetable extract immersed in boiling water or water from vegetables
Side dish of cold slaw, celery stalks or radishes or 1 artichoke

No. 9 (Tuesday)

Breakfast

2 ripe bananas peeled and sliced
1 apple, sliced
A small handful of raisins
Dressed with 2 tablespoons nut cream

Lunch

Combination Salad No. 13 with ½ cup almond cream
½ avocado

Dinner

1 plate cauliflower soup
Brussels sprouts, 1 onion and 2 peeled and sliced potatoes steamed in Savory Double Boiler
Dressed with 2 tablespoons flaxseed meal and vegetable extract immersed in hot water; dairy butter or a wholesome nut margarine may substitute
Side dish of watercress

No. 10 (Wednesday)

Breakfast

5 ounces dried Black Mission Figs (soaked in water over night and warmed in the morning)
Dressed with 2 tablespoons nut cream
1 ripe banana

Lunch

Combination Salad No. 16
2 whole wheat gems

Dinner

1 dish stewed lima beans or baked soy beans (6 ounces) with tomato sauce
½ head lettuce
⅓ cup grated carrots
Apply Plain Salad Dressing to salad

No. 11 (Thursday)

Breakfast

1 basket strawberries (about 10 ounces)
2 ripe bananas, peeled and sliced
Dressed with 2 tablespoons nut cream and tablespoon honey

Lunch

Combination Salad No. 17 with Plain Salad Dressing and cottage cheese
1 glass buttermilk

Dinner

Equal parts of string beans, asparagus, 1 sliced onion, steamed in Savory Double Boiler
Sour Cream Dressing
1 baked potato and butter or 2 potato cakes

No. 12 (Friday)

Breakfast

1 large orange or 2 medium sized ones
1 dozen dates
1 ounce shelled pecan nuts

Lunch

Combination Salad No. 18 with French Dressing
A few sun-dried olives or ½ avocado

Dinner

1 plate okra or string bean soup with radishes
2 slices (8 ounces) nut loaf with tomato sauce
A few sprigs of parsley and young green onions as a relish
1 artichoke

No. 13 (Saturday)

Breakfast

1 box raspberries
2 ripe bananas, peeled and sliced
Dressed with 2 tablespoons nut cream and 1 tablespoon honey

Lunch

Combination Salad No. 19 with mayonnaise
Whole rye wafers or 2 corn and potato muffins

Dinner

1 small head cauliflower, ½ bunch celery and 1 sliced onion steamed in Savory Double Boiler, mashed with butter and 1 poached egg
Relish of cold slaw and sliced turnips or rutabagas

No. 14 (Sunday)

Breakfast

1 pound cherries
1 ounce pecan or walnut meats

Lunch

Combination Salad No. 21 with Plain Salad Dressing and nut butter dressing
2 slices whole wheat bread with butter

Dinner

1 plate asparagus soup with radishes
2 slices pecan loaf with banana sauce or 2 slices soy bean loaf with tomato sauce
3 stalks stuffed celery, filled with minced vegetables and mayonnaise

SUMMER MENUS

No. 15 (Monday)

Breakfast

1 pound apricots pitted and cut in halves dressed with 2 tablespoons nut cream

Lunch

Combination Salad No. 9 with plain salad dressing and nut cream
2 whole wheat peanut gems

Dinner

2 slices of pignolia nut loaf (8 ounces) with rhubarb or tomato sauce
Steamed asparagus
1 dish of sliced cucumbers, garnished with celery stalks, radishes and ripe olives

No. 16 (Tuesday)

Breakfast

1 pound sliced peaches dressed with 2 tablespoons nut cream

Lunch

Combination Salad No. 10
2 summer squash halved and buttered

Dinner

2 artichokes steamed or 2 egg plants baked and halved
Apply ½ cup nut cream
Relish of ripe olives and pepper rings
1 or 2 ears of fresh sweet corn on cob, raw or slightly steamed

No. 17 (Wednesday)

Breakfast

1 orange
6 to 8 fresh figs, cut into halves and dressed with 2 tablespoons nut cream

Lunch

Combination Salad No. 11
1 glass soy bean milk (soy milk powder and honey may be diluted in water and served cold)

Dinner

Banana and apple pudding dressed with lemon sauce or Sunshine Salad (See page 161)
Stuffed Dates

No. 18 (Thursday)

Breakfast

1 pound fresh prunes or plums pitted and cut into halves; 1 ounce shelled pecan nuts or 2 tablespoons almond cream

Lunch

Combination Salad No. 12
Glass of buttermilk

Dinner

Carrot pudding No. 1 (10 to 12 ounces) with apple sauce
4 to 6 honey coconut macaroons or rolled oat macaroons

No. 19 (Friday)

Breakfast

1 box loganberries
2 ripe bananas peeled and sliced
Dressed with 2 tablespoons nut cream and 1 tablespoon honey

Lunch

Combination Salad No. 14
1 or 2 ears of fresh sweet corn on cob with butter

Dinner

Combination Salad No. 40
3 stalks celery stuffed with almond cream and dotted with raisins

No. 20 (Saturday)

Breakfast

½ grapefruit with teaspoon honey
3 or 4 medium-sized pears sliced and dressed with 2 tablespoons nut cream

Lunch

Combination Salad No. 32
2 Italian squash, halved lengthwise and buttered

Dinner

1 plate fruit salad No. 33
½ dozen stuffed dates
1 cup Irish Moss Custard

No. 21 (Sunday)

Breakfast

1 box blackberries
2 ripe bananas peeled and sliced
Dressed with 1 tablespoon honey and 2 tablespoons nut cream

Lunch

Combination Salad No. 15
Glass of buttermilk, if relished

Dinner

1 plate California fruit salad No. 34
1 cup nut cream custard
3 stalks celery

FALL MENUS

No. 22 (Monday)

Breakfast

1 pound seedless grapes
6 walnuts (1 ounce shelled)

Lunch

Combination Salad No. 20 with nut butter dressing
2 muffins

Dinner

1 plate Pear Salad No. 38
A few Stuffed Prunes or Raisin-Nut Balls (see page 149)

No. 23 (Tuesday)

Breakfast

2 peaches
1 slice watermelon
1 ounce shelled pecan nuts

Lunch

Combination Salad No. 22
2 slices steamed brown bread

Dinner

1 plate cream of grape soup
1 plate Raisin and Celery Salad No. 36 with grated nuts, or Peach and Melon Salad No. 44 with nut cream
3 or 4 honey coconut macaroons

No. 24 (Wednesday)

Breakfast

½ pound grapes
½ cantaloupe or slice of cassaba melon dressed with 2 tablespoons nut cream

Lunch

Combination Salad No. 23 with mayonnaise
2 slices whole wheat bread

Dinner

1 plate celery or vegetable soup with 4 whole wheat crackers
2 slices Savory Nut Loaf (about 8 ounces)
Side dish of sliced buttered beets
Side dish of watercress or endive

No. 25 (Thursday)

Breakfast

1 large pear
1 slice cassaba melon
6 walnuts (1 ounce shelled)

Lunch

Combination Salad No. 24 with Plain Salad Dressing and cottage cheese
1 slice banana squash

Dinner

3 walnut patties with cranberry sauce
Baked halved eggplant with butter
3 stalks celery stuffed with minced raw vegetables and mayonnaise
1 cup lemon gelatine

No. 26 (Friday)

Breakfast

1 pound muscat grapes
1 ounce shelled almonds

Lunch

Combination salad No. 25 with sour cream dressing
Glass of Soy Malted Milk or plain soy milk

Dinner

1 plate okra soup with whole wheat crackers
Carrot Pudding No. 2 (10 to 12 ounces)
1 dish jellied raw vegetables, jelled with agar or pectin

No. 27 (Saturday)

Breakfast

1 orange or apple
6 or 8 whole figs cut into halves, dressed with 2 tablespoons nut cream

Lunch

Combination salad No. 26, dressed with mayonnaise
Side dish of brussel sprouts creamed with nut butter or 1 artichoke

Dinner

1 plate string bean soup
Swiss chard (8 ounces), 2 sliced carrots and 1 large onion, steamed in double boiler
1 baked potato with butter

No. 28 (Sunday)

Breakfast

2 medium sized persimmons, sliced, dressed with 2 tablespoons almond cream

Lunch

1 plate of cream of tomato soup
Combination salad No. 27 with plain salad dressing and cottage cheese

Dinner

1 plate Tropical Salad No. 35
1 cup orange gelatine
6 stuffed dates

MENUS OF UNCOOKED FOODS

Winter Menus

No. 29

Breakfast

1 orange or ½ grapefruit with honey or
5 ounces unsulphured dried fruit, soaked in water over night and warmed in the morning, dressed with 2 tablespoons nut cream

Lunch

Choice of vegetable combination salads with stuffed celery
½ cup germinated wheat with seedless raisins ground together in food chopper (see instructions for germinated cereals)

Dinner

Combination fruit and nut salad consisting of
2 apples
2 ripe bananas
1 dozen dates or ½ cup seedless raisins
1 ounce shelled nuts
2 or 3 fruit and nut confections

Spring Menus

No. 30

Breakfast

Berry and banana combination No. 39 with nut cream

Lunch

Choice of vegetable combination salads with stuffed celery
½ cup germinated wheat or flaked wheat

Dinner

Choice of fruit combination salads
Choice of fruit and nut confections (about 3 ounces)

Summer Menus

No. 31

Breakfast

1 medium sized cantaloupe or ½ cassaba melon dressed with 2 tablespoons nut cream and 1 tablespoon honey

Lunch

Choice of vegetable combination salads
1 ear of fresh sweet corn

Dinner

Cherry and Banana salad No. 42 with almond cream
or Apricot and Banana salad No. 43 with nut cream
Choice of fruit and nut confections (3 ounces)

Fall Menus

No. 32

Breakfast

1 pound of any kind of table grapes
1 apple or 6 dates
1 ounce of shelled nuts

Lunch

Choice of vegetable combination salads
Unfired pumpkin pie or fresh sweet corn

Dinner

1 pound sliced persimmons or pears dressed with
2 tablespoons of almond cream or
Choice of fruit combination salads
Choice of fruit and nut confections (3 ounces)

The Change from a Cooked to a Raw Food Diet

Theoretically speaking, uncooked foods are superior to cooked foods, as they supply all the food constituents, especially the vitamins and mineral elements in their original intact condition. There is no doubt that people with perfect teeth and good digestive organs, having an opportunity for daily out-of-door exercise, can derive the fullest benefit from natural uncooked foods such as fruits, nuts, green leaf vegetables, supplemented occasionally by some dairy products. But there are a large number of people who have used all their lives mostly cooked foods, and through lack of regular outdoor exercise, have so weakened their organs of digestion and assimilation, that they cannot derive the greatest amount of nourishment from uncooked foods. For such people the change from the ordinary to a raw food diet should be gradual. Under present conditions for the majority of people, meals should consist of about 75 per cent natural, uncooked foods and 25 per cent properly prepared cooked foods. During Summer and Fall, when there is an abundance of fresh fruits and vegetables, the change in diet can be made without much difficulty.

CHAPTER XXII

ADULTERATION OF FOODS AND DRINKS

Due to the untiring efforts of the late Dr. Harvey W. Wiley, former chief of the Bureau of Chemistry, United States Department of Agriculture, the Federal Pure Food law was enacted by the Congress of the United States on June 30, 1906, and amended August 23, 1912, and March 3, 1913. On March 21, 1938 the President signed the Wheeler-Lea Act which broadens the powers of the former Federal Pure Food and Drug regulations. Before the passing of the Pure Food Law, the use of chemical preservatives and artificial colors was quite extensive, because it is not only cheaper to employ them than to preserve food by strictly hygienic methods, but inferior food materials can also be made more attractive and salable. The law still permits the use of certain preservatives and artificial colors, provided due notice is given to that effect on the labels of packages containing these substances. In other words, it is left to the often uninformed consumer himself to choose between natural and artificially colored and preserved foods.

Adulteration of foods and drinks, as generally understood, includes a number of injurious and deceptive practices. According to existing laws, food is regarded as adulterated if anything has been mixed with it to reduce its quality or strength; if anything inferior or cheaper has been substituted, wholly or in part; if it consists wholly or in part of a diseased, decomposed, or putrid animal or vegetable substance; if by coloring, coating, or otherwise, it is made to appear of greater value than it really is; if it contains any added poisonous ingredients, which include mineral and coal tar dyes and chemical preservatives (anti-ferments or antiseptics). Misbranding or mislabeling also constitute adulteration.

There has been an attempt made to divide preservatives into two classes; the first to be permitted (such as salt, saltpeter, sugar, vinegar and wood smoke), and the other class to be strictly forbidden (boric and salicylic acid and saccharine, as an artificial sweetener) Sodium benzoate and sulphur dioxide have only been partly restricted.

The New Federal Food and Drugs Act

The present act deals with the following items and is in many ways more stringent than were the previous rulings. *Adulteration of Food, Adulteration of Drugs, Adulteration of Cosmetics, Misbranding of Foods and Drugs, False Advertising, Tolerance for Poisonous Ingredients in Foods and Cosmetics and Certification of Coal Tar Colors for Food, Definitions and Standards for Food, Hair Dyes and Tonics, Remedies for Obesity and for Leanness, Curative Devices of All Sorts from Sun Lamps to Orthopaedic Shoes.*

Those who are interested in the details of the new law should write to the Secretary of Agriculture, Food and Drug Administration, Washington, D. C., for a copy.

Sodium Benzoate and Sulphur Dioxide

Sodium benzoate is largely used in the preservation of fruit juices, tomato catsup and oleomargarine. Sulphur dioxide is still permitted in limited amounts in the preparation of dried fruits, but the producers and packers are always inclined to go beyond the allowed minimum which is 0.35 parts of sulphur dioxide in one thousand parts of fruit. Many European countries have restricted the amount of sulphur in fruit to 1 part in 7,000. According to the investigations of Alfred W. McCann in New York City, the quantity of sulphur dioxide found by analysis in the 1923 pack of Calfornio dried fruits ranged all the way up to 3.5 parts per 1,000, which is ten times more than the law allows. The 1924 pack, the analysis of which was completed January, 1925, was practically identical in sulphur dioxide content with the pack of 1923. The remedy is in the consumer's hands. Let him see to it that he protects his own interests by demanding fruits free from sulphur dioxide.

Salt

Salt (chloride of sodium) has been employed in preparing and preserving food-stuffs for many centuries, although there is little physiological necessity for it. Natural foods, especially vegetables, if rationally prepared and grown on properly fertilized soil, furnish much of the necessary sodium and chlorine for proper nutrition. The following table gives the approximate amounts of salt per pound in some commonly used foods:

Food	Amount	Food	Amount
Bread	30 grains	Salt Ham	1/3 to 1 ounce
Cheese	1/3 to 1/2 ounce	Salt Beef	1 to 1½ ounces
Sauerkraut	1/3 to 1/2 ounce	Salt Pork	1½ to 1¾ ounces
Salt Butter	1/3 to 1 ounce	Salt Herring	1½ to 2 ounces
Smoked Sausage	1/2 to 1 ounce	Cod Liver Oil	2½ to 3 ounces

Common Table Salt is one of the most insidious condiments and preservatives because of its daily use by the great majority of people, despite the many clinical experiences which prove its injuriousness. The tendency of the average human mind is to find an excuse for its perverted habits, and to overlook and ignore the facts which are against its preconceived notions or desires. Those who will not dispense with salt entirely should at least see that the amount consumed daily does not exceed 25 grains, or as much as will go on the point of a knife. Yet there are many people who take an ounce and more per day, especially if they freely use salt butter and salt meat.

Condiments, Etc.

Although there is no law to regulate the use of salt, spices, especially pepper and vinegar, yet their extensive use in the preparation of our foods makes the latter unfit for the formation of healthy blood and tissues. Pepper and vinegar interfere with the formation of red blood corpuscles and through their constant irritating effect upon the mucous membranes of the intestinal canal, they are the chief contributory causes of chronic catarrh and cancer. Salted, pickled and spiced foods will insidiously lead to overeating and to the craving for alcoholic beverages. It has been truly said that cooks make more drunkards than do brewers, wine makers and distillers.

Saltpeter

Saltpeter, in addition to its preservative action, has the property of maintaining, as well as intensifying the red color of beef. Under the present law it has been ruled that saltpeter may be used pending further investigatons regarding its wholesomeness. Of course saltpeter, being an inorganic substance like coarse common salt, always impedes the vital functions of the body, as has been explained.

Boric Acid and Borax

Boric acid and borax, which are employed purely for their preservative effect, and sulphites, which act both to preserve and to give meat a bright appearance, are not permitted under the present United States meat inspection law. In England and Canada, on the other hand, no objection is made to the use of limited amounts of boric acid and borax.

Saccharine

Saccharine has been used as a substitute for sugar in many foods in which sugar is commonly recognized as a normal ingredient. The amendment of the Pure Food Law states that saccharine in foods is a deleterious ingredient, and that the substitution of saccharine for sugar in foods reduces and lowers their quality. Saccharine is often used by diabetics in place of sugar, but in every instance the drug will prove harmful to the patient.

Mineral and Coal Tar Dyes

Mineral dyes have been mostly replaced by coal tar dyes, with the exception of copper sulphate which is frequently used to preserve the color of vegetables and ripe olives. The law permits the use of any natural vegetable or animal color which is not injurious, but it is more stringent with regard to all artificial or synthetic colors. Only seven artificial colors have so far been authorized and of these the purity of each color must be attested before it can be used legally. Any coloring which is intended to mislead is illegal, and in most cases the fact that the food has been artificially colored must be plainly stated. Those who value their health will abstain from all products (candies, soft drinks, etc.) synthetically colored.

Laxity in the Enforcement of the Pure Food Law

Due to the political influence exerted by powerful commercial interests, there has developed some laxity in enforcing the Pure Food Law. The manufacturers of artificially colored and preserved foods generally have chemists in their employ who are always ready to testify in favor of their products, and to belittle their injurious effects. The argument generally made that small amounts of an injurious substance are not harmful is wholly untenable. It may be conceded that the occasional use of small quantities of preservatives is not dangerous, so far as producing any immediate fatality is concerned, but after continued use, they certainly are found injurious, as has been proved by many scientific experiments. In nearly all European countries the use of colors and preservatives in foods has been very much restricted by law.

As in the case of all poisons, the fact that the injurious effects of diminutive doses are not traceable at once, affords no proof that the continuous use of chemical preservatives is harmless. It is the constantly falling drop of water that finally disintegrates the rock. Any substance which prevents chemical action outside the body must naturally interfere with the processes of digestion and assimilation. Many chronic digestive troubles are due to the continuous use of preservatives. Carefully examine, therefore, the labels of all foods and drinks you buy and always select natural foods, guaranteed to be free from artificial colors and chemical preservatives.

SPRAYING OF FRUIT AND VEGETABLES WITH POISONOUS CHEMICALS

The loss of fruits and vegetables through insect pests in the United States amounts to about $300,000,000 every year. To combat these pests various poisonous chemical compounds in powdered and liquid form for spraying fruits and leaves are used. The principal spraying material are *Bordeaux mixture* (copper-sulphate of lime), *fluosilicate, calcium arsenate* and *lead arsenate.* The latter is mostly used on apples and pears.

To comply with government regulations, vegetables and fruit packing houses have installed washing machines where the various sprayed products are rinsed with water, containing about one per cent hydrochloric acid. However, there often remain traces of the spray on the fruit and the U. S. Department of Agriculture established the following tolerances: arsenic, .01 of a grain; lead 0.014, with no tolerance at all for fluorine. If the origin of green leaf vegetables and fruits cannot be ascertained by the consumer, it is advisable to give them an additional cleansing with a solution of hydrochloric acid (2 oz. to a gallon of water) before preparing them for the table. For this purpose a five gallon earthenware crock or large enameled dishpan should be used. Pour in a solution of two gallons of water and ½ cup of hydrochloric acid which may be purchased at any drug store. Fruits and vegetables should remain in this solution for about 3 minutes, then thoroughly drained and finally rinsed again in clean water to remove any traces of hydrochloric acid. The solution should be renewed after 3 days of use.

The advantage of raising vegetables and fruits in the home garden on properly mineralized soil, as outlined in the chapter on soil culture, becomes apparent. Rational soil culture will greatly reduce the breeding of insects and prevent some of the enormous losses from which agriculture is suffering today, at the same time improving the quality and durability of the food products.

APPENDIX

TABLES OF ANALYSES

Explanation of the Tables of Analyses

The amounts of organic salts in 1000 parts of water-free substance have been calculated by the author with the object of furnishing a means of comparing them on an equal basis with the respective amounts of total mineral matter contained in the solid material. Where no figures are given no analysis was available.

Analyses of mineral matter of different foods, grown in different localities should be made frequently, in order to determine the variation of their mineral contents and the particular elements needed for improving both soil and food products. This is highly important, when we consider the fact that many plant diseases and insect pests are traceable to impoverished or wrongly fertilized soils.

The analyses presented in these tables have been taken mostly from the following sources:

Dr. J. Koenig, *Chemie der Menschlichen Nahrungs und Genussmittel* (Chemistry of Human Foods and Food-Accessories).

Dr. E. Wolff, *Aschen Analysen* (Analyses of Mineral Matter in Foods).

Dr. Ragner Berg, *Die Nahrungs und Genussmittel, ihre Zusammensetzung, und ihr Einfluss auf die Gesundheit mit besonderer Beruecksichtigung der Aschen Bestandteile* (Foods, their Composition and Influence upon Health, with Special Reference to their Contents of Mineral Matter).

Dr. Henry C. Sherman, *Chemistry of Food and Nutrition.*

U. S. Department of Agriculture, Bureau of Chemistry, Bulletin No. 87, *Chemical Composition of Some Tropical Fruits and their Products.*

Wilson Popenoe, *Manual of Tropical and Subtropical Fruits.*

Bulletins published by Professor E. P. Forbes of the Ohio Agricultural Experiment Station.

As life originated in the sea which contains nearly all the known elements, we may assume that many other elements, besides those mentioned in the tables are connected with the various life-processes. The spectroscope reveals the presence of at least forty elements in living protoplasms. The following have been identified, although some of them in exceedingly small quantities:

Aluminum
Argon
Arsenic
Beryllium
Boron
Bromine
Cerium
Chromium
Cobalt
Copper
Fluorine
Helium
Iodine
Lanthanum
Lead
Lithium
Manganese
Molybdemium
Neodymium
Neon
Nickel
Rubidium
Scandium
Strontium
Titanium
Vanadium
Zinc

As it has been explained in Chapter IX these rarer elements may be obtained in an organic form from the vegetation of the sea. There are two kinds of sea plants which have been lately prepared in a dehydrated and powdered form for human consumption, viz: *Kelp* (Macrocystis Pyrifera) and *Dulse* (Rhodymenia Palmata). These may be used daily with much benefit in place of the inorganic table salt.

BERRIES AND DECIDUOUS FRUITS	AVERAGE CHEMICAL COMPOSITION PER CENT					COMPOSITION OF MINERAL MATTER IN 1,000 PARTS OF WATER FREE SUBSTANCE — ACID BINDING ELEMENTS						ACID FORMING ELEMENTS			
	WATER	PROTEIN	FAT	CARBOHYDRATES	MINERAL MATTER	TOTAL	POTASSIUM K_2O	SODIUM Na_2O	CALCIUM CaO	MAGNESIUM MgO	IRON Fe_2O_3	PHOSPHORUS P_2O_5	SULPHUR SO_3	SILICON SiO_2	CHLORINE
APPLES	84.80	0.40	0.50	13.00	0.50	33.00	11.78	8.61	1.35	2.89	0.46	4.52	2.01	1.42	.....
APRICOTS	84.70	1.42	.....	13.34	0.54	33.60	19.68	3.76	1.08	1.12	0.26	3.76	0.92	2.80	0.20
BLACKBERRIES	86.30	1.30	1.00	10.90	0.45	40.15	17.90	0.60	7.95	4.75	0.05	6.20	0.90	.....	1.80
CHERRIES, average	79.80	1.00	0.80	16.70	0.70	34.60	17.94	0.76	2.60	1.90	0.70	5.54	1.76	3.11	0.48
CRANBERRIES	88.90	0.40	0.60	8.40	0.40	36.00	9.00	0.03	10.15	0.90	0.04	1.60	14.20	.....	0.03
CURRANTS, red	82.20	0.30	.....	11.30	0.45	25.00	12.10	0.04	1.46	0.95	0.03	2.17	7.95	.....	0.35
CURRANTS, white	81.20	0.40	.....	13.60	0.44	23.50	16.90	0.16	0.29	0.45	0.05	1.40	3.95	.....	0.30
CURRANTS, black	76.80	1.00	.....	18.70	0.51	22.30	13.70	0.13	0.60	0.75	0.04	2.27	4.73	.....	0.08
GOOSEBERRIES	85.70	0.50	.....	8.40	0.40	29.00	11.22	2.87	3.54	1.70	1.32	5.71	1.71	0.75	0.22
GRAPES, average	78.20	1.30	1.25	18.60	0.65	30.00	18.75	0.40	2.70	1.25	0.45	4.00	1.50	0.60	0.35
HUCKLEBERRIES	78.40	0.80	0.60	16.60	1.00	46.30	26.44	3.00	3.70	2.82	0.50	8.05	1.44	0.42	.....
MEDLAR	74.60	0.50	0.30	16.50	0.60	.....	.....	.....	.....	.....	.....	.....	.....	.....	.....
MIRABELLES	80.90	0.60	.....	13.60	0.46	24.25	13.50	1.80	1.40	1.20	0.35	4.80	1.05	.....	0.15
MULBERRIES	84.70	0.40	.....	14.30	0.60	.....	.....	.....	.....	.....	.....	.....	.....	.....	.....
MUSKMELONS	89.50	0.60	.....	7.20	0.60	.....	.....	.....	.....	.....	.....	.....	.....	.....	.....
NECTARINES	82.90	0.60	.....	15.90	0.60	.....	.....	.....	.....	.....	.....	.....	.....	.....	.....
PEARS	84.40	0.60	0.50	14.10	0.40	25.60	14.00	2.17	2.05	1.52	0.25	3.90	1.45	0.38	.....
PEACHES	88.10	0.70	0.10	9.40	0.48	40.70	20.90	3.00	4.60	1.35	0.50	6.05	3.50	.....	0.80
PLUMS	78.40	1.00	.....	20.00	0.60	27.80	16.45	0.15	2.78	1.53	0.90	4.17	1.03	0.68	.....
PRUNES, average	81.20	0.80	.....	16.50	0.70	37.75	18.28	3.41	4.34	1.36	0.94	6.03	1.21	1.19	0.15
PRUNES, French	80.50	0.90	.....	18.50	0.60	30.00	20.95	0.92	0.90	1.60	0.25	3.47	0.64	1.35	0.07
RASPBERRIES, black	84.10	1.70	1.00	12.60	0.60	.....	.....	.....	.....	.....	.....	.....	.....	.....	.....
RASPBERRIES, red	85.80	1.00	.....	9.70	0.60	42.25	16.50	1.90	3.15	1.75	0.05	4.50	11.50	.....	2.90
STRAWBERRIES	87.70	1.00	0.60	7.70	0.80	65.00	13.72	18.53	9.23	.....	3.73	7.97	2.05	7.83	1.10
WATERMELONS	92.50	0.50	0.20	6.70	0.30	40.00	18.00	3.75	4.00	2.10	1.75	5.60	2.10	1.60	1.10

TROPICAL AND SUBTROPICAL FRUITS	AVERAGE CHEMICAL COMPOSITION PER CENT					COMPOSITION OF MINERAL MATTER IN 1,000 PARTS OF WATER FREE SUBSTANCE — ACID BINDING ELEMENTS						ACID FORMING ELEMENTS			
	WATER	PROTEIN	FAT	CARBOHYDRATES	MINERAL MATTER	TOTAL	POTASSIUM K_2O	SODIUM Na_2O	CALCIUM CaO	MAGNESIUM MgO	IRON F_2O_3	PHOSPHORUS P_2O_5	SULPHUR SO_3	SILICON SiO_2	CHLORINE
AVOCADO	70.55	2.10	20.00	6.00	1.35	45.00	11.75	8.35	2.15	2.36	0.67	8.00	5.05	0.22	6.45
BANANAS	75.30	1.30	0.60	22.00	0.80	32.40	16.10	5.60	0.68	2.40	0.07	2.85	1.20	0.80	2.70
BREADFRUIT	73.10	1.57	0.51	14.60	1.15	42.75	17.50	2.10	6.30	0.50	trace	5.10	3.75	....	1.50
CACTUS LEAVES	94.66	0.72	0.09	3.30	1.23	....	....	....	....	....	....	....	....	....	....
CACTUS FRUIT	79.20	1.40	1.30	11.70	2.70	....	....	....	....	....	....	....	....	....	....
CHERIMOYA	72.13	....	....	9.16	1.04	37.00	18.40	....	0.81	0.25	....	2.43	1.67	....	2.74
DATES, average	20.00	2.10	2.80	70.00	1.60	20.00	10.50	1.00	1.15	1.19	0.06	1.00	1.20	....	3.90
DURIAN	55.50	2.30	....	23.70	1.24	....	....	....	....	....	....	....	....	....	....
FEIJOA	83.87	1.02	0.05	11.16	0.45	....	....	....	....	....	....	....	....	....	....
FIGS, black, fresh	79.00	1.50	0.20	18.70	0.60	....	....	....	....	....	....	....	....	....	....
FIGS, black, dried	20.00	5.50	1.00	63.00	3.20	40.00	10.50	9.60	3.50	3.40	0.60	6.30	2.70	2.40	1.00
FIGS, SMYRNA, dried	18.80	4.30	0.30	74.20	2.40	29.30	17.10	0.90	3.30	1.68	0.66	3.85	1.20	....	0.61
GRAPEFRUIT	86.90	0.56	....	7.37	0.39	30.00	13.20	....	2.20	1.20	0.38	3.32	1.00	....	0.40
GUAVAS	82.90	1.30	0.70	8.00	0.50	29.40	15.47	....	0.75	0.48	....	2.44	1.05	0.30	1.55
GUAVAS, strawberry	79.42	0.76	0.95	8.05	0.77	....	....	....	....	....	....	....	....	....	....
JUJUBE	68.10	1.44	0.21	21.66	0.73	....	....	....	....	....	....	....	....	....	....
LEMONS	89.30	1.00	0.70	8.50	0.50	46.70	22.54	0.84	12.75	2.09	0.20	5.25	1.25	0.31	0.18
LIMES	85.15	0.83	....	0.58	0.98	66.00	28.38	....	5.17	1.56	....	5.70	2.24	....	2.65
LITCHI, fresh	79.08	1.15	0.20	15.30	0.54	....	....	....	....	....	....	....	....	....	....
LITCHI, dried	16.04	2.90	0.80	78.00	1.90	....	....	....	....	....	....	....	....	....	....
LOQUATS	77.90	0.20	....	20.20	1.10	....	....	....	....	....	....	....	....	....	....
MANGO	87.40	0.60	0.40	9.90	0.50	40.00	18.95	....	2.55	0.64	....	2.60	1.47	....	1.55
OLIVES, dried	30.07	5.24	51.90	10.45	2.34	33.40	27.02	2.52	2.50	0.06	0.30	0.46	0.36	0.22	0.06
ORANGES, average	86.90	0.80	0.20	11.60	0.50	38.15	18.62	0.95	8.65	2.03	0.38	4.70	2.00	0.25	0.29
PAPAYA	87.80	0.50	0.05	10.30	0.56	....	....	....	....	....	....	....	....	....	....

TROPICAL AND SUBTROPICAL FRUITS	AVERAGE CHEMICAL COMPOSITION PER CENT					COMPOSITION OF MINERAL MATTER IN 1,000 PARTS OF WATER FREE SUBSTANCE — ACID BINDING ELEMENTS						ACID FORMING ELEMENTS			
	WATER	PROTEIN	FAT	CARBOHYDRATES	MINERAL MATTER	TOTAL	POTASSIUM K_2O	SODIUM Na_2O	CALCIUM CaO	MAGNESIUM MgO	IRON Fe_2O_3	PHOSPHORUS P_2O_5	SULPHUR SO_3	SILICON SiO_2	CHLORINE
PAWPAW	76.60	5.20	0.90	16.80	0.50	....	....	....	....	....	....	....	....	....	....
PERSIMMON	66.10	0.80	0.70	29.70	0.90	....	....	....	....	....	....	....	....	....	....
PINEAPPLE	89.30	0.40	0.30	9.70	0.30	28.60	12.55	2.20	3.10	2.10	0.40	1.40	4.15	....	2.70
POMEGRANATE	76.80	1.50	1.60	16.80	0.60	25.90	8.00	12.25	1.65	0.90	0.06	2.50	0.20	....	0.34
SAPODILLA	75.00	0.87	0.55	20.00	1.00	....	....	....	....	....	....	....	....	....	....
SAPOTE, white	74.74	0.87	0.55	21.75	0.47	....	....	....	....	....	....	....	....	....	....
SOUR SOP	80.00	1.65	0.50	14.00	0.86	....	....	....	....	....	....	....	....	....	....
SWEET SOP	75.12	1.53	0.54	18.15	0.80	....	....	....	....	....	....	....	....	....	....
STAR APPLE	88.50	2.35	1.38	4.40	0.40	....	....	....	....	....	....	....	....	....	....
TAMARIND	47.50	1.36	....	31.43	1.56	....	....	....	....	....	....	....	....	....	....
DRIED FRUITS															
APPLES	26.10	1.60	2.20	62.00	2.00	....	....	....	....	....	....	....	....	....	....
APRICOTS	29.40	4.70	1.00	62.50	2.40	....	....	....	....	....	....	....	....	....	....
PEARS	16.50	2.80	5.40	66.00	2.40	....	....	....	....	....	....	....	....	....	....
PEACHES	20.00	3.15	0.45	50.00	2.15	....	....	....	....	....	....	....	....	....	....
PRUNES	22.30	2.10	....	71.20	2.30	30.00	19.15	0.80	1.40	1.75	0.80	4.20	0.80	0.90	0.10
RAISINS	14.60	2.60	3.30	73.60	3.40	40.00	19.40	3.30	2.45	2.30	0.60	7.30	2.55	....	2.10
CURRANTS (Zante)	17.20	2.40	1.70	74.20	4.50	54.35	30.00	3.15	1.60	1.85	0.30	12.40	3.10	....	1.75

NUTS	AVERAGE CHEMICAL COMPOSITION PER CENT					COMPOSITION OF MINERAL MATTER IN 1,000 PARTS OF WATER FREE SUBSTANCE — ACID BINDING ELEMENTS						ACID FORMING ELEMENTS			
	Water	Protein	Fat	Carbohydrates	Mineral Matter	Total	Potassium K_2O	Sodium Na_2O	Calcium CaO	Magnesium MgO	Iron Fe_2O_3	Phosphorus P_2O_5	Sulphur SO_3	Silicon SiO_2	Chlorine
Acorns, dried	4.10	8.10	37.40	48.00	2.40	25.00	16.30	0.15	1.80	1.30	0.25	3.70	1.05		0.45
Almonds	4.90	21.40	54.40	16.80	2.50	26.30	5.23	0.38	3.04	3.95	0.23	10.10	0.96	0.04	0.06
Beechnuts	9.09	21.70	42.50	19.20	3.86	42.00	7.20	2.18	7.73	5.94	0.42	12.81	1.03	1.13	1.03
Brazil Nuts	4.70	17.40	65.00	5.70	3.30	34.60	6.65	0.37	6.10	2.90	0.10	13.30	4.33		0.85
Butternuts	4.50	27.90	61.20	3.40	3.00										
Candlenuts	5.90	21.40	61.70	4.90	3.30										
Chestnuts, dried	5.90	10.70	7.00	74.20	2.20	23.40	11.40	0.28	1.07	1.87	0.14	5.50	3.00	0.04	0.01
Chufa (Earth Almond)	2.20	3.50	31.60	60.70	2.00										
Cocoanut	14.10	5.70	50.60	27.90	1.70	22.80	9.75	1.30	1.10	1.30	0.40	4.80	0.85		3.20
Cocoanut, desiccated	3.50	6.30	57.40	31.50	1.30										
Cocoanut Milk	92.70	0.40	1.50	4.60	0.80										
Filberts	5.40	16.50	64.00	11.70	2.40	25.25	6.65	0.20	3.60	1.98	0.46	7.30	4.46		0.60
Hickory Nuts	3.70	15.40	67.40	11.40	2.10										
Paradise Nuts	2.30	22.20	62.60	10.20	2.70										
Pecans	3.40	12.10	70.70	8.50	1.60	16.60	5.80	0.36	1.33	2.20	0.23	6.75			
Pinons	3.40	14.60	61.90	17.30	2.90	30.00	5.70	0.75	2.62	4.20	0.60	13.15			
Pignolias, Italian	6.20	33.90	48.20	7.90	3.80										
Pistachios	4.20	22.60	54.50	15.60	3.10										
Walnuts, Black	2.50	27.60	56.30	11.70	1.90										
Walnuts, English	2.50	18.40	64.40	13.00	1.70	17.40	2.20	0.17	0.97	2.88	0.61	10.10	0.22	0.12	0.12
Water Chestnuts	12.30	4.00	1.20	50.00	1.77	20.02	12.30	trace	0.90	1.15	trace	5.10	0.45		0.15
Peanuts	7.40	29.80	43.50	14.70	2.25	24.30	9.27	0.21	0.95	2.29	0.27	10.60	0.45	0.05	0.23
Peanut Butter	2.10	29.30	46.50	17.10	2.20										
Almond Butter	2.20	21.70	61.50	11.60	3.00										

VEGETABLES	AVERAGE CHEMICAL COMPOSITION PER CENT					COMPOSITION OF MINERAL MATTER IN 1,000 PARTS OF WATER FREE SUBSTANCE — ACID BINDING ELEMENTS						ACID FORMING ELEMENTS			
	WATER	PROTEIN	FAT	CARBOHYDRATES	MINERAL MATTER	TOTAL	POTASSIUM K_2O	SODIUM Na_2O	CALCIUM CaO	MAGNESIUM MgO	IRON Fe_2O_3	PHOSPHORUS P_2O_5	SULPHUR SO_3	SILICON SiO_2	CHLORINE
ARTICHOKES	79.24	1.80	0.14	16.70	1.10	53.00	25.32	5.38	1.75	1.55	2.00	7.40	2.60	5.30	2.06
ASPARAGUS	93.75	1.80	0.25	2.60	0.54	86.40	20.94	14.77	9.33	3.72	2.94	16.07	5.36	9.50	5.10
BEETS	87.50	1.60	0.10	9.70	1.10	88.00	38.70	9.00	5.45	2.73	0.26	8.27	6.15	7.90	9.00
BEETS, red	88.00	1.20	0.20	10.10	0.50	41.65	8.45	21.60	2.50	0.10	1.00	2.55	0.50	2.00	2.95
BRUSSELS SPROUTS	85.60	3.50	0.30	6.80	1.37	95.40	31.40	0.35	2.40	2.35	0.60	20.25	35.30	.....	2.75
CABBAGE	90.00	1.90	0.20	4.80	1.23	123.00	45.38	11.68	21.65	4.90	0.86	11.07	17.10	1.10	10.45
CABBAGE, red	90.06	1.83	0.20	5.86	0.77	77.00	17.00	9.33	21.48	3.41	0.08	3.00	9.58	0.38	10.51
CABBAGE, Savoy	87.10	3.30	0.70	6.00	1.64	127.00	34.80	12.95	27.17	8.13	2.16	18.63	10.41	6.07	10.03
CARROTS	87.05	1.00	0.20	9.40	0.90	69.00	25.46	14.63	7.80	3.04	0.70	8.83	4.45	1.66	3.18
CAULIFLOWER	90.90	2.50	0.30	4.55	0.83	91.20	40.46	5.38	5.10	3.37	0.91	18.42	11.86	3.37	3.10
CELERY	94.50	1.10	0.10	3.30	1.00	180.00	48.60	65.25	14.70	6.75	1.60	14.50	6.50	4.30	17.80
CELERY ROOT	84.10	1.50	0.40	11.80	0.84	52.80	22.70	trace	6.90	3.05	0.75	6.75	2.95	2.10	8.45
CHICORY ROOT	78.80	0.80	0.20	18.30	0.73	32.85	13.20	5.05	2.40	1.60	0.85	4.30	2.70	.....	2.75
CHIVES	82.00	2.80	0.50	10.00	0.95	53.00	18.05	2.28	11.27	2.90	0.80	8.12	6.66	.....	2.32
COLLARDS	87.10	4.50	0.60	6.30	1.50	.....	.....	.....	.....	.....	.....	.....	.....	.....	.....
CUCUMBERS	95.60	1.20	0.10	2.30	0.44	100.00	41.20	10.00	7.30	4.15	1.40	20.20	6.90	8.00	6.60
DANDELION	85.50	2.80	0.70	7.45	1.90	131.00	50.95	13.63	26.20	11.00	1.10	10.22	2.88	9.17	3.47
DILL	83.80	3.50	0.90	7.30	2.40	142.00	28.70	12.65	31.95	11.55	1.00	20.30	20.05	2.40	14.75
EGGPLANT	92.90	1.20	0.30	5.10	0.50	70.00	39.05	2.80	3.05	4.20	0.25	9.50	4.45	.....	6.70
GARLIC	64.70	6.80	0.10	27.90	1.50	.....	.....	.....	.....	.....	.....	.....	.....	.....	.....
HORSERADISH	76.70	2.70	0.35	16.00	1.50	64.40	19.81	2.57	5.28	1.87	1.25	4.96	19.84	8.18	8.18
JERUSALEM ARTICHOKE	79.10	1.50	0.10	17.00	1.05	50.00	26.20	5.80	1.80	1.60	2.15	7.65	2.70	....	2.10
KALE	93.80	1.90	0.10	3.00	1.58	255.00	81.50	5.35	28.10	7.30	1.30	35.50	86.00	.....	10.50
KOHLRABI	85.90	4.90	0.20	8.20	1.17	83.00	29.30	5.40	9.15	5.65	2.50	1.70	7.35	2.05	4.10
LEEK, bulbs	87.60	2.80	0.30	6.50	1.24	100.00	30.70	14.15	10.40	2.90	7.60	16.70	7.40	7.40	3.10
LEEK, leaves	90.80	1.50	0.30	5.10	0.69	75.70	33.25	5.55	17.70	3.60	0.50	6.25	3.35	.....	5.50

VEGETABLES	AVERAGE CHEMICAL COMPOSITION PER CENT					COMPOSITION OF MINERAL MATTER IN 1,000 PARTS OF WATER FREE SUBSTANCE — ACID BINDING ELEMENTS						ACID FORMING ELEMENTS			
	WATER	PROTEIN	FAT	CARBOHYDRATES	MINERAL MATTER	TOTAL	POTASSIUM K_2O	SODIUM Na_2O	CALCIUM CaO	MAGNESIUM MgO	IRON Fe_2O_3	PHOSPHORUS P_2O_5	SULPHUR SO_3	SILICON SiO_2	CHLORINE
LETTUCE	94.30	1.40	0.30	2.20	1.03	180.70	67.94	13.55	26.56	11.20	9.40	16.62	6.87	14.64	13.82
LETTUCE, Romaine	92.50	1.54	0.43	4.20	1.33	177.60	44.90	62.70	21.10	7.60	2.30	19.40	6.90	5.30	7.40
LETTUCE, Lambs'	93.40	2.70	0.40	2.70	0.79	120.00	53.00	11.20	7.20	2.60	0.45	10.20	5.80	24.00	5.70
OKRA	90.20	1.60	0.20	7.40	0.60	61.35	8.80	12.00	21.00	3.30	trace	9.00	7.10	.....	.....
ONIONS	87.60	1.60	0.30	9.90	0.60	48.40	12.10	1.55	10.65	2.55	2.20	7.25	2.65	8.10	1.35
PARSLEY	85.05	3.70	0.70	7.45	1.70	.....	.....	.....	.....	.....	.....	.....	.....	.....	.....
PARSNIPS	83.00	1.60	0.50	13.50	1.40	80.20	33.80	0.32	4.80	2.50	0.25	10.25	8.00	9.60	10.40
PEPPER, green	92.00	1.10	0.10	4.60	1.00	.....	.....	.....	.....	.....	.....	.....	.....	.....	.....
POTATOES	75.00	2.08	0.15	21.00	1.10	44.20	26.56	1.33	1.15	2.18	0.48	7.47	2.89	0.88	1.55
POTATOES, sweet	69.00	1.80	0.70	27.40	1.10	35.50	18.60	2.20	3.10	0.85	0.50	2.20	1.05	1.40	5.50
PUMPKINS	90.30	1.10	0.13	6.50	0.70	72.15	13.85	15.22	5.55	2.45	1.88	23.80	1.73	5.27	0.30
RADISH, large	86.90	1.90	0.10	7.40	1.07	82.30	18.00	3.05	6.60	2.85	1.00	33.70	6.35	6.75	4.00
RADISH, small	93.30	1.20	0.15	3.80	0.74	110.50	35.10	23.15	16.30	3.35	3.00	12.00	7.15	1.00	10.00
RHUBARB	94.40	0.60	0.70	3.60	0.70	125.00	74.50	6.45	12.55	.....	1.84	18.41	2.34	3.46	6.81
RUTABAGAS	88.90	1.30	0.20	8.50	1.10	100.00	46.30	13.60	8.80	5.20	1.70	18.10	5.30	.....	1.00
SALSIFY	85.40	4.30	0.30	6.80	1.20	.....	.....	.....	.....	.....	.....	.....	.....	.....	.....
SALSIFY, black	80.40	1.00	0.50	17.10	1.00	48.80	15.30	6.40	3.40	2.07	1.48	12.95	5.60	.....	1.60
SORREL	92.20	1.70	0.30	3.90	0.98	125.80	56.05	0.85	7.00	8.70	9.85	21.35	13.30	.....	8.70
SPINACH	88.50	3.50	0.60	4.44	2.10	182.60	29.90	63.90	21.50	11.50	6.05	18.05	12.45	8.10	11.30
SUGARBEETS	81.30	1.00	0.10	15.80	0.70	37.40	20.15	3.35	2.30	3.00	0.45	4.60	1.60	.....	1.85
SUGARBEET LEAVES	88.75	1.91	0.03	8.64	0.70	63.60	23.40	11.00	15.60	7.35	0.40	3.25	2.60	.....	.....
SWISS CHARD	92.50	1.54	0.43	4.20	1.33	177.60	44.90	62.70	21.70	7.60	2.30	19.40	6.90	5.30	7.40
TOMATOES	94.00	0.90	0.20	3.75	1.05	175.00	82.50	32.90	11.35	13.55	1.00	10.75	5.00	1.75	18.00
TURNIPS	89.90	3.50	0.10	11.30	1.28	126.00	59.10	7.10	14.24	4.66	0.75	18.27	12.10	1.40	8.30
TURNIP LEAVES	.....	.....	.....	.....	.....	.....	22.63	8.16	27.39	2.78	1.29	3.71	4.38	.....	.....
WATER CRESS	92.30	1.90	0.10	1.30	1.46	190.00	44.75	17.25	35.00	8.60	0.35	22.40	53.90	.....	7.75

CEREALS BREADS ETC.	AVERAGE CHEMICAL COMPOSITION PER CENT					COMPOSITION OF MINERAL MATTER IN 1,000 PARTS OF WATER FREE SUBSTANCE									
						ACID BINDING ELEMENTS						ACID FORMING ELEMENTS			
	WATER	PROTEIN	FAT	CARBOHYDRATES	MINERAL MATTER	TOTAL	POTASSIUM K_2O	SODIUM Na_2O	CALCIUM CaO	MAGNESIUM MgO	IRON Fe_2O_3	PHOSPHORUS P_2O_5	SULPHUR SO_3	SILICON SiO_2	CHLORINE
BARLEY, whole	13.80	11.10	2.20	64.90	2.70	31.30	8.80	1.05	1.10	3.70	0.40	15.00	0.70	0.20	0.35
BARLEY, pearled	11.50	8.50	1.10	77.80	1.10	12.30	2.70	0.40	0.22	0.80	0.22	5.20	2.40	....	0.35
BUCKWHEAT	13.27	11.41	2.68	68.79	2.38	27.45	6.32	1.68	1.21	3.41	0.47	13.35	0.55	0.06	0.35
CORN, yellow, whole	13.10	9.85	4.60	68.50	1.51	18.50	5.50	0.20	0.36	2.87	0.15	8.44	0.15	0.39	0.35
CORN MEAL, bolted	12.60	7.10	1.30	78.40	0.60	6.85	2.50	0.02	0.13	1.02	0.10	3.08	....	....	....
CORN, green (on the cob)	75.40	3.10	1.10	19.20	0.70	28.45	8.50	3.20	0.50	2.65	0.07	8.28	3.68	0.50	1.12
CORN, popped	4.30	10.70	5.00	77.30	1.30	....	....	....	....	....	....	....	....	....	....
CORN, Egyptian	14.30	10.06	3.29	68.35	2.03	....	....	....	....	....	....	....	....	....	....
CORN, Kaffir	9.30	9.90	3.00	74.90	1.50	....	....	....	....	....	....	....	....	....	....
CORN, Milo Maize	9.00	10.70	2.80	72.20	2.30	....	....	....	....	....	....	....	....	....	....
MILLET	11.50	9.00	3.80	70.25	1.95	22.00	4.46	0.71	0.28	3.26	0.42	13.00	....	1.60	....
OATS, whole	12.40	10.40	5.20	57.80	3.02	34.50	10.40	1.35	2.25	4.25	0.40	14.30	0.80	0.40	0.35
OATMEAL	7.30	16.05	7.20	67.50	1.95	20.00	5.50	1.00	1.10	1.75	0.05	8.10	1.40	0.20	1.10
OATS, rolled	7.70	16.70	7.30	66.20	2.10	22.60	6.50	1.30	1.50	2.10	0.60	7.15	1.45	0.20	0.60
RICE, whole	13.10	7.85	0.88	76.50	1.00	16.00	3.60	0.67	0.59	1.78	0.22	8.60	0.10	0.40	0.02
RICE, polished	12.55	7.90	0.52	77.80	0.35	4.00	0.87	0.22	0.13	0.45	0.05	2.15	0.03	0.11	0.01
RICE, bran	12.90	11.10	7.85	62.10	4.55	52.30	6.00	....	1.35	9.15	4.00	22.85	0.12	8.85	....
RYE, whole	15.06	11.50	1.80	67.80	1.81	21.30	6.84	0.31	0.61	2.39	0.25	10.16	0.28	0.30	0.01
RYE, flour, bolted	12.90	6.80	0.90	78.70	0.70	8.00	2.75	0.15	0.10	0.60	0.15	3.35	....	....	....
RYE, bran	10.90	17.40	3.70	69.06	5.00	56.10	15.75	0.75	1.95	8.80	1.40	26.70	....	1.15	....
SORGHUM	12.80	9.10	3.60	69.80	2.10	24.00	6.00	0.90	0.35	5.20	0.58	10.60	0.12	....	0.25
WHEAT, whole, average	13.40	13.60	1.90	69.10	2.00	23.10	7.20	0.50	0.75	2.80	0.30	10.90	0.09	0.46	0.07
WHEAT, white flour	12.60	10.20	0.90	74.70	0.50	5.70	1.82	0.08	0.43	0.44	0.03	2.80	....	....	....
WHEAT, middlings	11.73	15.22	4.77	60.55	2.85	....	....	....	....	....	....	....	....	....	....
WHEAT, bran	12.40	16.60	3.50	62.10	4.85	55.00	15.15	0.33	1.65	9.35	0.38	27.80	0.13	0.50	....
WHEAT, germ	12.50	35.70	13.10	31.20	5.70	....	....	....	....	....	....	....	....	....	....

CEREALS BREADS ETC.	AVERAGE CHEMICAL COMPOSITION PER CENT					COMPOSITION OF MINERAL MATTER IN 1,000 PARTS OF WATER FREE SUBSTANCE									
						ACID BINDING ELEMENTS						ACID FORMING ELEMENTS			
	WATER	PROTEIN	FAT	CARBOHYDRATES	MINERAL MATTER	TOTAL	POTASSIUM K_2O	SODIUM Na_2O	CALCIUM CaO	MAGNESIUM MgO	IRON Fe_2O_3	PHOSPHORUS P_2O_5	SULPHUR SO_3	SILICON SiO_2	CHLORINE
BREAD, whole wheat	35.70	8.90	1.80	52.10	1.50	23.30	4.15	4.10	1.55	1.05	0.30	4.75	0.60	....	6.80
BREAD, white	35.30	9.20	1.30	53.10	1.10	17.00	1.50	4.90	0.40	0.48	0.03	3.20	1.80	....	4.70
PUMPERNICKEL	42.20	4.20	0.70	43.30	1.35	23.30	2.35	6.40	1.50	2.35	0.45	4.50	0.85	....	4.80
SWEDISH RYE CRISP	8.10	8.00	0.60	70.10	1.95	21.20	5.60	2.70	1.00	1.20	0.08	5.85	2.90	....	1.90
SAGO	12.20	9.00	0.40	78.10	0.30	N. B. The large amount of Sodium and Chlorine in									
TAPIOCA	11.40	0.40	0.10	88.00	0.10	Bread is caused by the addition of table salt.									
OILY SEEDS—															
CARAWAY SEED	13.15	19.84	18.73	7.65	5.85	67.35	17.75	4.40	12.05	5.55	2.35	16.25	3.65	3.30	2.05
MUSTARD SEED	7.18	27.59	29.66	20.83	4.47	48.15	7.80	2.90	8.75	5.05	0.50	19.25	2.40	1.20	0.25
POPPY SEED	7.50	19.40	38.40	12.80	4.27	46.10	6.27	0.46	16.30	4.50	0.18	14.48	0.74	1.52	2.12
SUNFLOWER SEED	7.50	14.20	32.30	14.50	3.50	37.80	6.12	2.80	2.87	4.65	0.60	13.38	0.87	5.54	0.90
FLAX SEED	9.20	22.60	33.70	26.89	4.30	....	....	....	....	....	....	....	....	....	....
HEMP SEED	8.90	18.20	32.60	21.10	4.20	....	....	....	....	....	....	....	....	....	....
SESAME	5.30	35.99	24.62	22.83	7.42	....	....	....	....	....	....	....	....	....	....
STARCHY ROOTS															
SWEET CASSAVA	66.00	1.10	0.20	30.20	0.70	....	....	....	....	....	....	....	....	....	....
TARO	70.90	1.80	0.20	23.20	1.20	....	....	....	....	....	....	....	....	....	....
YAMS	72.90	1.80	0.20	23.30	0.90	....	....	....	....	....	....	....	....	....	....
YAUTIA TUBERS	70.00	2.20	0.20	26.10	0.90	....	....	....	....	....	....	....	....	....	....
EDIBLE FUNGI—															
MUSHROOMS	89.10	2.60	0.30	6.10	0.70	64.20	32.68	1.05	0.65	2.18	1.02	21.60	2.50	0.65	0.57
CHAMPIGNONS	91.30	3.74	0.15	3.50	0.50	74.70	37.87	1.27	0.55	0.37	0.85	11.50	18.15	1.05	3.45
TRUFFLES	77.60	7.70	0.50	6.60	1.92	83.30	31.50	1.50	8.15	1.05	4.65	27.65	5.00	0.20	1.10

LEGUMES	AVERAGE CHEMICAL COMPOSITION PER CENT					COMPOSITION OF MINERAL MATTER 1000 PARTS OF WATER FREE SUBSTANCE CONTAIN — ACID BINDING ELEMENTS						ACID FORMING ELEMENTS			
	WATER	PROTEIN	FAT	SUGAR, STARCH	MINERAL MATTER	TOTAL	POTASSIUM K_2O	SODIUM Na_2O	CALCIUM CaO	MAGNESIUM MgO	IRON Fe_2O_3	PHOSPHORUS P_2O_5	SULPHUR SO_3	SILICON SiO_2	CHLORINE
BEANS, dried	14.76	24.30	1.60	49.00	3.26	38.20	15.85	0.42	1.91	2.73	0.19	14.86	1.30	0.25	0.69
BEANS, Blackeye	8.48	21.43	1.28	61.28	4.78	....	....	....	....	....	....	....	....	....	4.78
CHICK PEAS (Garbanzas)	14.80	13.00	1.60	51.50	3.76	44.25	8.10	0.40	1.45	18.35	0.80	13.10	1.10	....	0.95
COW PEAS, dried	13.00	21.40	1.40	60.80	3.40	39.10	21.00	2.40	1.50	3.15	....	6.85	3.60	....	0.60
HORSE BEANS	14.00	18.00	0.50	50.50	2.75	32.00	15.25	0.40	0.15	0.30	0.10	14.30	1.15	....	0.60
KIDNEY BEANS, dried	13.60	23.12	2.28	53.63	3.53	40.85	18.00	0.58	2.60	3.00	0.13	14.30	1.65	0.23	0.34
KIDNEY BEANS, green	84.10	3.90	0.20	8.30	0.70	44.00	23.30	1.70	2.75	1.65	0.05	5.65	7.00	....	1.90
LENTILS	12.35	25.70	1.90	53.30	3.04	34.70	11.60	4.60	2.10	0.90	0.60	12.20	1.20	....	1.50
LIMA BEANS, dried	10.40	18.10	1.50	65.90	4.10	45.00	27.60	4.10	1.25	3.10	0.01	6.10	2.60	....	0.04
LIMA BEANS, green	68.50	7.10	0.70	22.00	1.70	54.00	33.90	4.75	1.40	3.60	0.14	6.60	3.10	....	0.50
PEAS, dried	15.00	22.85	1.80	52.40	2.58	30.03	13.06	0.30	1.45	2.42	0.24	10.87	1.03	1.27	0.53
PEAS, green	74.60	7.00	0.50	16.90	1.00	39.50	15.40	1.10	1.60	2.80	0.04	11.20	6.00	....	1.40
ST. JOHN'S BREAD	17.30	5.70	1.10	67.00	2.50	....	....	....	....	....	....	....	....	....	....
SOY BEANS	10.75	34.00	16.80	33.70	4.75	53.22	24.65	0.60	3.45	3.45	0.28	17.50	2.65	0.27	0.40
STRING BEANS, fresh	84.10	3.90	0.20	8.30	1.20	75.00	32.00	1.75	7.50	6.25	0.05	6.50	12.75	....	7.10
MISCELLANEOUS—															
HONEY	18.20	0.40	....	81.20	0.20	2.80	0.02	0.10	2.35	0.01	0.12	0.18	0.01	....	0.01
RAW SUGAR	2.16	0.30	....	94.60	0.96	9.80	5.97	1.30	0.70	0.03	0.04	0.03	0.95	....	0.78
SUGAR CANE	75.40	1.50	0.53	21.82	0.70	28.40	....	....	....	....	....	....	....	....	....
MOLASSES	25.10	2.40	....	69.30	3.20	42.70	27.00	0.38	4.22	1.36	0.02	0.88	2.58	....	6.34
COCOA BEANS	3.60	12.00	49.30	26.40	3.50	36.00	12.96	0.82	1.95	4.00	0.02	13.95	1.25	0.55	0.30
COCOA	6.30	21.50	27.30	31.60	5.20	....	....	....	....	....	....	....	....	....	....
CHOCOLATE	3.60	2.40	20.00	58.50	1.55	16.80	6.14	0.13	1.00	3.20	0.03	4.80	0.95	....	0.55
MAPLE SYRUP	27.00	....	....	71.40	0.39	5.35	2.80	0.13	1.43	0.45	0.04	0.20	0.07	....	0.13
OLEOMARGARINE	9.10	0.50	84.50	....	1.65	18.10	0.60	6.70	....	....	....	0.40	....	....	10.40

MILK (HUMAN AND ANIMAL) AND DAIRY PRODUCTS	AVERAGE CHEMICAL COMPOSITION PER CENT					COMPOSITION OF MINERAL MATTER IN 1,000 PARTS OF WATER FREE SUBSTANCE — ACID BINDING ELEMENTS						ACID FORMING ELEMENTS			
	WATER	PROTEIN	FAT	CARBOHYDRATES	MINERAL MATTER	TOTAL	POTASSIUM K_2O	SODIUM Na_2O	CALCIUM CaO	MAGNESIUM MgO	IRON Fe_2O_3	PHOSPHORUS P_2O_5	SULPHUR SO_3	SILICON SiO_2	CHLORINE
HUMAN	87.75	1.60	3.95	6.25	0.45	34.70	11.73	3.16	5.80	0.75	0.07	7.84	0.33	0.07	6.38
COW'S	87.30	3.55	3.70	4.88	0.71	55.50	13.70	5.34	12.24	1.69	0.30	15.79	0.17	0.02	8.04
DOG'S	75.60	11.20	9.60	3.10	1.35	55.30	5.70	3.25	18.20	0.80	0.08	19.75	0.25	0.15	6.55
SWINE'S	82.30	5.90	6.90	3.80	1.10	65.00	9.35	6.95	21.35	1.20	0.25	16.20	0.30	0.25	9.15
SHEEP'S	80.80	6.50	6.90	4.90	0.90	47.40	5.03	4.65	11.70	2.15	0.17	17.70	0.20	0.10	5.70
GOAT'S	85.70	4.30	4.50	4.40	0.80	70.00	15.60	3.45	13.90	2.30	0.60	21.05	0.30	0.20	13.50
MARE'S	91.50	1.30	1.20	5.70	0.41	48.20	12.05	1.60	14.25	1.50	0.20	15.00	0.15	0.05	3.55
RABBIT'S	69.40	15.50	10.50	2.00	2.60	85.00	11.40	7.75	33.60	1.75	0.07	22.80	0.40	0.30	7.00
BUFFALO'S	82.20	4.40	7.10	4.70	0.85	48.00	6.60	2.88	15.95	1.50	0.08	16.15	1.37	.....	3.47
CAMEL'S	87.10	3.60	2.70	5.30	0.75	58.15	10.50	2.00	15.48	2.70	0.12	17.20	2.05	.....	8.10
COW BUTTER	11.00	1.00	85.00	.....	3.00	33.70	1.75	12.10	0.90	0.18	0.05	0.12	6.85	.....	11.75
BUTTERMILK	90.00	3.00	0.50	4.80	0.70	77.00	18.10	8.50	14.40	2.60	0.60	21.80	1.30	.....	9.70
CREAM	74.00	2.50	18.50	4.50	0.50	19.20	5.15	1.55	4.25	0.60	0.50	3.90	0.45	.....	2.00
SKIM MILK	90.50	3.40	0.30	5.10	0.70	73.70	22.60	7.10	15.20	2.20	0.60	13.40	2.40	.....	10.20
WHEY	93.80	0.60	0.07	5.10	0.44	71.00	21.85	9.75	13.65	0.25	0.40	12.00	1.90	.....	11.20
CONDENSED MILK	68.20	9.60	9.30	11.20	1.70	.....	.....	.....	.....	.....	.....	.....	.....	.....	.....
COTTAGE CHEESE	72.50	20.90	1.00	4.30	1.25	45.00	5.40	0.90	14.35	1.00	0.30	15.35	0.60	.....	7.10
CHEESE, average	38.80	23.75	30.00	1.50	4.50	73.50	2.70	17.90	27.60	1.10	0.04	20.20	7.76	.....	26.20
EGGS, whole	73.70	12.55	12.10	0.55	1.10	41.80	6.27	9.56	4.56	0.46	0.17	15.72	0.13	0.13	3.72
WHITE OF EGGS	85.75	12.70	0.25	0.70	0.60	42.10	13.21	13.30	1.18	1.18	0.25	1.85	0.88	0.45	12.08
YOLK	50.80	16.20	31.95	0.10	1.10	24.40	2.70	1.44	3.17	0.51	0.40	15.22	.....	0.21	0.45
SEA FOODS——															
CRABS	77.10	16.60	2.00	1.20	3.10	.....	.....	.....	.....	.....	.....	.....	.....	.....	.....
MUSSELS	84.20	8.70	1.10	4.10	1.90	.....	.....	.....	.....	.....	.....	.....	.....	.....	.....
SHRIMPS	70.80	25.40	1.00	0.20	2.60	.....	.....	.....	.....	.....	.....	.....	.....	.....	.....

HUMAN BODY AND ANIMAL FOODS	AVERAGE CHEMICAL COMPOSITION PER CENT					COMPOSITION OF MINERAL MATTER 1,000 PARTS OF WATER FREE SUBSTANCE CONTAIN										
							ACID BINDING ELEMENTS					ACID FORMING ELEMENTS				
	WATER	PROTEIN	FAT	CARBOHYDRATES (SUGAR, STARCH)	MINERAL MATTER	TOTAL	POTASSIUM K_2O	SODIUM Na_2O	CALCIUM CaO	MAGNESIUM MgO	IRON Fe_2O_3	PHOSPHORUS P_2O_5	SULPHUR SO_3	SILICON SiO_2	CHLORINE	FLUORINE
HUMAN BODY, whole	60.00	19.00	15.00	1.00	5.00	125.00	3.30	3.00	70.50	2.15	0.70	32.15	4.10	1.00	7.00	1.10
RED BLOOD CORPUSCLES	68.78	30.20	.....	.....	1.02	35.00	13.82	5.87	0.55	0.30	5.00	3.50	0.28	trace	5.68	.....
BLOOD PLASMA	90.00	9.00	.....	0.15	0.85	85.00	3.30	36.75	3.20	2.35	.....	1.75	1.45	0.22	36.20	.....
BLOOD SERUM	90.75	8.24	.....	0.15	0.86	94.50	3.60	41.80	3.50	2.45	.....	1.60	1.55	0.22	40.00	.....
LYMPH	94.00	4.00	0.40	0.05	0.73	121.60	3.93	57.88	1.17	0.31	0.06	1.32	.....	0.50	54.75	.....
LUNGS	80.00	15.20	3.65	.....	1.90	95.00	1.24	24.70	1.80	3.04	0.30	46.07	1.32	0.36	6.17	.....
BRAIN	80.60	8.50	9.30	.....	1.10	56.70	19.50	6.80	0.40	0.70	0.16	27.30	0.42	0.07	4.35	.....
LIVER	71.55	20.00	3.65	3.25	1.55	54.50	13.90	7.90	1.97	0.11	1.44	27.30	0.50	0.14	1.26	.....
SPLEEN	75.50	17.10	4.20	1.00	1.56	63.80	6.12	28.26	4.77	0.30	4.64	17.26	1.55	0.11	0.35	.....
BILE	86.00	.....	.....	.....	0.85	60.00	2.88	30.35	0.85	0.32	0.14	6.27	3.83	0.21	15.06	.....
FRESH BONES	(Dry fat free substance)					650.00	.....	.....	240.00	8.00	10.00	345.00	.....	.....	12.00	15.00
FRESH MUSCLE TISSUE	75.50	18.70	3.70	1.00	1.10	49.00	18.00	2.80	0.40	1.80	0.20	22.00	0.60	0.40	2.80	.....
BLOOD OF BULLOCKS	80.80	18.10	0.20	0.05	0.85	44.30	3.29	19.80	0.48	0.26	4.14	2.31	1.34	0.35	15.14	.....
BLOOD OF CALF	83.56	15.20	0.13	0.30	1.09	70.30	7.15	27.00	1.18	0.80	5.46	5.10	0.76	.....	22.90	.....
BLOOD OF SHEEP	79.80	19.02	0.18	0.20	0.98	52.00	3.45	22.00	0.56	0.30	4.70	2.70	0.90	.....	17.45	.....
BLOOD OF HOG	76.89	22.23	0.19	.....	0.79	36.20	8.00	10.00	0.45	0.46	3.04	4.15	0.35	.....	9.75	.....
MEAT, average	72.00	20.00	5.00	0.40	1.10	40.00	16.65	1.44	1.12	1.28	0.15	17.00	0.64	0.44	1.56	.....
BEEF	76.00	18.00	5.00	.....	1.00	41.70	15.24	2.70	0.08	1.00	0.18	7.02	3.10	.....	2.35	.....
PORK	75.00	20.25	6.80	.....	0.72	29.10	9.37	5.76	0.30	1.03	.....	7.86	3.02	.....	1.77	.....
CHICKEN	72.20	21.30	4.55	0.75	0.90	32.85	14.72	3.00	0.35	1.17	.....	8.00	3.70	.....	1.90	.....
SEA FISH, average	80.00	18.00	0.80	.....	1.20	60.00	18.55	4.50	1.50	2.00	0.05	23.50	3.40	.....	6.50	.....
PIKE	79.60	17.90	0.50	.....	1.22	60.00	14.80	12.00	4.50	2.25	.....	23.00	0.55	.....	2.90	.....
SALMON, fresh	64.00	20.05	12.30	.....	1.77	49.15	8.70	4.90	3.10	3.40	0.40	17.30	3.75	.....	7.60	.....
OYSTERS, fresh	86.90	6.20	1.20	3.70	1.47	116.50	6.70	34.10	3.80	2.75	0.30	11.50	13.00	.....	44.50	.....
CLAMS	85.80	8.60	1.00	2.00	2.60	.....	.....	.....	.....	.....	.....	.....	.....	.....	.....	.....
LOBSTER	79.20	16.40	1.80	0.40	2.20	.....	.....	.....	.....	.....	.....	.....	.....	.....	.....	.....

SODIUM (Na_2O)

Contained in 1000 parts of water-free substance

White Flour	0.08	Sorghum	0.90	Apricots	3.76	Pike	12.00
Honey	0.10	Oranges	0.95	Chives	4.20	Dill	12.65
Chocolate	0.13	Dates	1.00	Sea Fish	4.50	Savoy Cabbage	12.95
Maple Sugar	0.13	Oatmeal	1.00	Lentils	4.62	White of Eggs	13.30
Rye Flour, bolted	0.15	Mushrooms	1.05	Salmon	4.90	Lettuce	13.55
Walnuts	0.17	Barley	1.05	Cow's Milk	5.34	Dandelions	13.63
Peanuts	0.21	Champignons	1.27	Artichokes	5.38	Leeks	14.15
Chestnuts	0.28	Cocoanuts	1.30	Cauliflower	5.38	Carrots	14.63
Wheat Bran	0.33	Rolled Oats	1.30	Kohlrabi	5.40	Asparagus	14.77
Pecans	0.36	Raw Sugar	1.30	Beans	5.60	Pumpkins	15.22
Almonds	0.38	Beechnuts	2.17	Red Blood Corpuscles	5.87	Strawberries	18.53
Barley, pearled	0.38	Pears	2.18	Turnips	7.10	Radishes	23.37
Grapes	0.40	Olives	2.52	Chicken Meat	8.20	Lungs	24.70
Beans	0.42	Horseradish	2.57	Apples	8.01	Spleen	28.26
Whole Wheat	0.50	Gooseberries	2.87	Avocado	8.35	Bile	30.35
Filberts	0.65	Huckleberries	3.00	Beets	9.00	Tomatoes	32.90
Whole Rice	0.67	Currants, Zante	3.15	Red Cabbage	9.33	Oysters	34.10
Rye Bran	0.75	Human Milk	3.16	Whole Egg	9.56	Blood Plasma	36.75
Cherries	0.76	Corn, Green	3.20	Whey	9.75	Blood Serum	41.80
Cocoabeans	0.82	Nettles	3.28	Cucumbers	10.00	Lymph	57.88
Lemons	0.84	Raisins	3.30	Dried Figs	10.77	Swiss Chard	62.70
Sorrel	0.85	Prunes	3.41	Cabbage	11.68	Spinach	63.90
Cottage Cheese	0.90	Watermelons	3.75			Celery	65.25

CALCIUM (CaO)

Contained in 1000 parts water-free substance

Food	CaO	Food	CaO	Food	CaO	Food	CaO	Food	CaO
White Bread	0.10	Barley, whole	1.10	Beans	1.91	Blood Serum	3.50	Kohlrabi	9.15
Rye Flour, bolted	0.10	Cocoanut	1.10	Rye Bran	1.95	Gooseberries	3.54	Strawberries	9.23
Rice, polished	0.13	Oatmeal	1.10	Filberts	2.05	Huckleberries	3.70	Asparagus	9.33
Cornmeal, bolted	0.20	Meat, average	1.12	Pears	2.05	Oysters	3.80	Leek Bulbs	10.40
Barley, pearled	0.22	Dates	1.15	Avocado	2.15	Watermelons	4.00	Onions	10.65
Sorghum	0.35	Potatoes	1.15	Lentils	2.18	Molasses	4.22	Cow's Milk	12.24
Corn	0.36	White of Egg	1.18	Mushrooms	2.18	Prunes	4.34	Lemon	12.75
White Flour	0.43	Buckwheat	1.21	Oats, whole	2.25	Pike	4.50	Whey	13.65
Red Blood Corpuscles	0.55	Pecans	1.33	Honey	2.35	Whole Egg	4.56	Turnips	14.24
Whole Rice	0.59	Apples	1.35	Raisins	2.45	Parsnips	4.80	Cottage Cheese	14.35
Whole Rye	0.61	Rice Bran	1.35	Olives	2.50	Cauliflower	5.10	Radishes	15.45
Bananas	0.68	Chicken Meat	1.40	Pineapples	2.50	Tomatoes	5.20	Poppy Seed	16.30
Raw Sugar	0.70	Maple Syrup	1.43	Mango	2.55	Horseradish	5.28	Chives	20.70
Whole Wheat	0.75	Peas	1.45	Cherries	2.60	Pumpkins	5.55	Swiss Chard	21.10
Guavas	0.75	Cowpeas	1.50	Pine Nuts	2.62	Human Milk	5.88	Red Cabbage	21.48
Peanuts	0.95	Pumpernickel	1.50	Grapes	2.70	Bread Fruit	6.30	White Cabbage	21.65
Walnuts	0.97	Rolled Oats	1.50	Brazilnuts	2.75	Celeriac	6.90	Spinach	22.73
Chocolate	1.00	Sea Fish	1.50	Plums	2.78	Sorrel	7.00	Dandelions	26.20
Rye Crisp	1.00	Whole Wheat Bread	1.55	Almonds	3.04	Cucumbers	7.30	Lettuce	26.56
Chestnuts	1.07	Currants, Zante	1.60	Salmon	3.10	Beechnuts	7.73	Savoy Cabbage	27.17
Apricots	1.08	Wheat Bran	1.65	Yolk of Egg	3.17	Carrots	7.80	Dill	31.95
		Artichokes	1.75	Blood Plasma	3.20	Truffles	8.15	Water Cress	35.00
				Figs	3.30	Oranges	8.65	Nettles	38.58

IRON (Fe_2O_3)

Contained in 1000 parts water-free substance

Chicken	trace	Almonds	0.23	Whey	0.40	Mushrooms	1.02
Pike	trace	Pecans	0.23	Oats	0.41	Dandelions	1.18
Pork	trace	Peas	0.24	Millets	0.42	Horseradish	1.25
Cocoabeans	0.02	Acorns	0.25	Grapes	0.45	Gooseberries	1.32
Molasses	0.02	White of Egg	0.25	Apples	0.46	Rye Bran	1.40
Chocolate	0.03	Pears	0.25	Buckwheat	0.47	Cucumbers	1.40
White Flour	0.03	Rye	0.25	Brazil Nuts	0.50	Chives	1.50
Maple Syrup	0.04	Parsnips	0.25	Huckleberries	0.50	Watermelons	1.75
Cheese	0.04	Apricots	0.26	Barley	0.53	Pumpkins	1.88
Sea Fish	0.05	Beets	0.26	Figs	0.60	Artichokes	2.00
Polished Rice	0.05	Peanuts	0.27	Raisins	0.60	Savoy Cabbage	2.16
Dates	0.06	Cottage Cheese	0.30	Walnuts	0.61	Onions	2.20
Bananas	0.07	Oysters	0.30	Avocado	0.67	Swiss Chard	2.30
Human Milk	0.07	Pineapples	0.30	Lentils	0.69	Asparagus	2.94
Red Cabbage	0.08	Currants, Zante	0.30	Cherries	0.70	Radishes	3.00
Whole Corn	0.10	Cow's Milk	0.30	Carrots	0.70	Strawberries	3.73
Honey	0.12	Whole Wheat	0.30	Celeriac	0.75	Rice Bran	4.00
Chestnuts	0.14	Filberts	0.35	Turnips	0.75	Truffles	4.65
Meat, average	0.15	Wheat Bran	0.38	Chickpeas	0.80	Red Blood Corpuscles	5.00
Corn	0.15	Oranges	0.38	Cabbage	0.86	Spinach	6.05
Whole Egg	0.17	Barley	0.40	Champignons	0.88	Nettles	6.57
Poppy Seed	0.18	Yolk of Egg	0.40	Plums	0.90	Leeks	7.60
Beans	0.19	Salmon, fresh	0.40	Cauliflower	0.91	Lettuce	9.40
Lemons	0.20	Beechnuts	0.40	Prunes	0.94	Sorrel	9.85
Pearled Barley	0.22	Cocoanut	0.40	Dill	1.00	Hematin, red coloring matter of the blood	66.50
Whole Rice	0.22	Pineapple	0.40	Tomatoes	1.00		

INDEX

A

B

C

INDEX

D

INDEX

E

F

G

INDEX

INDEX

INDEX

INDEX

Q

R

S

INDEX

T

INDEX

INDEX